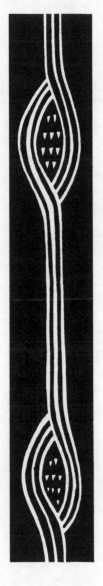

Braindance

DEAN FALK

A John Macrae Book

Henry Holt and Company   New York

Henry Holt and Company, Inc.
Publishers since 1866
115 West 18th Street
New York, New York 10011

Henry Holt® is a registered
trademark of Henry Holt and Company, Inc.

Copyright © 1992 by Dean Falk
All rights reserved.
Published in Canada by Fitzhenry & Whiteside Ltd.,
195 Allstate Parkway, Markham, Ontario L3R 4T8.

Library of Congress Cataloging-in-Publication Data
Falk, Dean.
Braindance / by Dean Falk.—1st ed.
p. cm.
"A John Macrae book."
Includes bibliographical references and index.
1. Australopithecines. 2. Fossil man. 3. Brain—Evolution.
4. Human evolution. I. Title.
GN283.F35 1992   91-14628
569'.9—dc20   *CIP*

ISBN 0–8050–1282–6
ISBN 0–8050–3186–3 (An Owl Book: pbk.)

Henry Holt books are available for special promotions and premiums.
For details contact: Director, Special Markets.

First published in hardcover in 1992 by Henry Holt and Company, Inc.
First Owl Book Edition—1994

DESIGNED BY PAULA R. SZAFRANSKI

Printed in the United States of America
All first editions are printed on acid-free paper. ∞

10 9 8 7 6 5 4 3 2 1
10 9 8 7 6 5 4 3 2 1 (pbk.)

*For my daughters Sarah Eve and
Adrienne Jane, and my granddaughters
Eve Penelope and Helen Dean*

Acknowledgments

I am grateful to many people for their help with this book. Jack Macrae has been a patient and encouraging editor, and special thanks is due Rebecca Holland (production editor at Henry Holt) for her extensive help with the manuscript. I thank Bill Calvin and John Brockman for their encouragement, advice, and help. Joyce Crocker envisioned and sketched the introductory illustrations for each chapter, and a number of the technical drawings were provided by Kathleen Addario. I am particularly pleased to have John Reader's beautiful photographs of fossil hominids in *Braindance*. (For other photographs, see the 1988 paperback edition of Reader's *Missing Links: The Hunt for Earliest Man*, Penguin Books.) Curt Busse is gratefully acknowledged for providing photographs of chimpanzees.

Kathleen Gibson and Tim Ingold invited me to participate in the Wenner-Gren sponsored International Symposium on Tools, Language and Intelligence: Evolutionary Implications, in Cascais, Portugal, during March 1990. In October of 1990, I attended another conference in Memphis, Tennessee, on "Laterality: Evolution and Mechanisms" that was organized by Jeannette Ward. Both conferences greatly influenced my thinking about hominid brain evolution and I am grateful to their organizers. The chapter "Taung Goes to St. Louis" could not have been written without the support of my wonderful collaborators at Washington University in St. Louis: Michael Vannier, Jim Cheverud, and Charles Hildebolt. I am also indebted to the National Science Foundation and the National Institutes of Health for supporting our research.

A number of other people provided helpful discussion, advice, and/or illustrations: Este Armstrong, Bob Brain, Michel Cabanac, Glenn Conroy, Elisabeth Davis, Irwin Flashman, Lauren Gage, Gordon Gallup, Stanley Glick, Roland Guay, Terry Harrison, Melissa Hines, Harry Jerison, Adam Kendon, Roger Lewin, John Pfeiffer, Cynthea Riffle, Amy Robbins, Sue Savage-Rumbaugh, Denise Schmandt-Besserat, Judy Torel, Russell Tuttle, Alan Walker, Michael Zansky, Adrienne Zihlman, and Betty Zimmerberg.

During the course of my undergraduate and graduate education, I was extremely fortunate to have three mentors who nurtured my development as a physical anthropologist and paleoneurologist. Although they should not be held responsible for the opinions expressed in this book, were it not for the guidance and inspiration of Charles A. Reed, C. Loring Brace, and the late Leonard Radinsky, *Braindance* would never have been written.

Contents

Introduction   1

1 Foraging in the Red Cave   9

2 Taung Goes to St. Louis   39

3 Chimp Brain, Human Brain   53

4 Of Family Trees, Darwin's Theory, and the Origins of Bipedalism   77

5 Boy Brain, Girl Brain   101

6 Lucy's Child: Mix-up at the Hospital   125

7 The Radiator Theory of Brain Evolution   151

8 Braindance   175

9 Brainwar   199

Notes and References   221

Index   249

Braindance

Introduction

Approximately five million years ago, a group of apelike individuals moved away from their relatives and began evolving in an independent direction that would one day allow their descendants to become human beings. This remarkable event occurred in East Africa, and early on, these ancestors of ours started walking on two legs. At that point these creatures with long arms, hairy skins, and large canines ceased to be apes and became the first hominids, known today as "australopithecines."

Charles Darwin's 1859 publication of *On the Origin of Species* sparked what would become an arduous controversy between creationists and evolutionists about the origin of human beings. Half a century later, many scientists and some of the public had reconciled their religious beliefs with the theory of natural selection and had even begun to apply that theory to the question of human origins. Yet many people still had difficulty with the notion of missing links and, in particular, the idea that we are descended from apelike ancestors. (The wife of England's Bishop of Worcester put it this way in 1860 after a much publicized debate about human evolution: "Descended from the apes! Let us hope it is not true, but if it is, let us pray that it will not become

1

generally known.") This attitude prevailed in the United States as late as 1925, when John Scopes was convicted of a crime for teaching evolutionary theory to high school students in Tennessee.

In a now-classic paper published that same year, a South African anatomist named Raymond Dart announced the discovery of the first australopithecine, a fossilized hominid child from a place called Taung. Dart's specimen seemed to reveal a mixture of apelike and humanlike features. Given the anti-intellectual climate within which Dart interpreted his find, it is perhaps not surprising that he overemphasized the humanlike attributes of his small fossil and downplayed its apelike qualities. At that time, people were probably more likely to accept a humanlike rather than an apelike ancestor, and it is possible that this fact subconsciously influenced early efforts to interpret early hominids.

Dart and his colleagues established what has become a long tradition of overemphasizing and overinterpreting the *humanlike* features of Taung and the other australopithecine fossils eventually discovered nearby. Even today, there are Old Guard paleoanthropologists who insist that australopithecines were more humanlike than apelike, especially in the refinement of their bipedalism, the development of their teeth, and the morphology of their brains. New investigators—this writer included—are applying recently developed measurement techniques to the study of australopithecine fossils. These studies show that Dart's australopithecines were far more apelike than was previously believed.

This is not to say that all scientists agree with that assessment and that advocacy has been removed from the study of hominid paleontology. Far from it! Controversies rage over technical matters, and scientists must decide, for example, which has greater value for evolutionary studies—direct examination of the fossil record or comparative studies of molecules of living species? Similarly, is it better to reckon the evolutionary relationships between different groups on the basis of special features whose functions may or may not be known (cladistic analysis) or by comparing the evolution of whole integrated physiological systems in these groups (functional morphology)? Yet, although evolutionary biologists may quibble mightily about such technical details, they all share a conceptual framework that is grounded in Darwinian theory. Their theoretical differences of opinion eventually get resolved by scientific means, despite the uninformed yelps of delight from creationists who assume that such differences invalidate evolutionary theory.

Clearly, there is much dispute over theoretical interpretation of the hominid fossil record. Paleoanthropologists believe that bipedalism provided a major impetus for the origin of hominids, but delineation of its causes is one of the hottest topics (and biggest mysteries) in hominid paleontology. The assumption that males were the primary focus of selection for various good and noble human features has also come under recent fire. As illustrated by an ongoing debate about the relative importance of man the hunter versus woman the gatherer, the recent convergence of sexual politics with paleoanthropology is having an important impact on how scientists interpret our origins. However, these controversies are nothing compared with those that ensue when investigators staunchly defend their prize fossils or their published hominid family trees—no matter what the evidence. In fact, this is happening right now in the case of a fossil called Lucy.

One reason why hominid paleontology is so contentious is because it is very much like an Old Boys club. To study fossils, you've got to be *privy* to them. Somebody has to let you into the shop. But the shop, alas, is a fairly closed one. Just a few people in the world control access to the fossils that must be studied if one is to do the research necessary to understand our origins. Unfortunately, published descriptions of newly discovered fossils are sometimes delayed (and the specimens withheld from colleagues) in anticipation of "publication by press conference" complete with spin control. It is tough for independent workers, whose scientific contributions are frequently ignored (and I am not only thinking of myself) if they conflict with the ideas of established authorities. If an outsider *does* succeed in getting new ideas published and discussed, he or she had better have a sturdy hide.

Lest I sound too petulant, I am pleased to say this book is less about the politics of paleoanthropology than it is about hominid brain evolution. It is also offered as an example of the exception that proves the rule. I was lucky enough to be allowed into an inner sanctum in South Africa to study casts of the interior of fossil skulls (endocasts) that reflect the brain's anatomy. To my surprise, these endocasts clearly indicated that the cerebral cortex of australopithecines was apelike, rather than humanlike, as had been believed since Dart's initial publication on the Taung fossil. Although my observations were documented and innocent of preconceived ideas, upon their publication I found myself plunged into what would become a decade-long bitter controversy.

Because australopithecine brains appeared apelike, it was necessary to investigate other early hominids to learn something about the evolution of the human brain. I therefore turned my attention to the fossil record of *Homo*, which goes back just two million years. And what a record it is. Not only did humanlike cerebral cortices first appear in early *Homo*, but the growth in brain size took off so fast that by the time of *Homo sapiens*, it had doubled. Why did brain size increase so dramatically in *Homo*, but not in the australopithecines? And what about the relationship between bipedalism and brain evolution? It used to be thought that the two were linked. Mary Leakey's spectacular discovery of fossilized footprints of early hominids that lived 3.5 million years ago shows that this was not the case. The makers of the footprints had clearly been bipedal, walking upright long before brain size began its dramatic increase in *Homo*. Why, then, did bipedalism precede the increase in brain size? I attempt an answer, the radiator theory of brain evolution, which you will encounter in this book.

But there is more to studying brain evolution than just looking at skulls and endocasts. Much can be gleaned from comparing the brains and cognitive capacities of humans with those of our closest nonhuman relatives, the chimpanzees. Comparative psychologists show us that chimpanzees are smart. Some chimps have even been taught nonverbal language. However, unlike most children, no chimpanzee has ever looked at its human caretaker and asked the question, Where do I come from? Chimpanzees are intelligent, but they simply do not have brains that are capable of formulating abstract questions.

Although the cerebral cortex of humans is larger and more convoluted than that of chimpanzees, human and chimp brains appear superficially to have the same parts. Thus, it appears that subtle differences in the nervous systems of humans and chimpanzees, not gross anatomy, are what count. These involve, in particular, the wiring and the distribution of neurochemicals in the frontal lobes and association cortices, as well as the right/left contrasts in brain organization, called lateralization.

The evolution of brain lateralization that occurred over the last two million years must have been especially important because modern humans depend on the left side of the brain for functions related to spoken language and right-handedness and on the right side of the brain for other abilities such as comprehending maps and composing music. Because these skills are unique in humans, it was believed until quite recently that humans were the only primates with lateralized brains. However, thanks to the dazzling work of investigators studying the nervous systems of rodents, birds, and nonhuman primates, it is now apparent that brain lateralization is the rule, rather than the exception, for a large variety of animals. The lateralized skills that appear to be uniquely human are actually derived from the less-lateralized calling, singing, and dexterity systems of our primate ancestors. Thus, although the extent of brain lateralization in humans is dramatic, it represents an end product on an evolutionary continuum rather than an evolutionary leap. A second myth is that the brains of men and women are exactly the same. This misconception is also being put to rest, due largely to recent breakthrough research on the effects of sex hormones on the brain. This book provides an evolutionary model that attempts to elucidate the ongoing evolution of brain lateralization in hominids while taking into account gender differences in the nervous system.

During the past two million years the dramatic increase in brain size in *Homo* was not only accompanied by subtle shifts in the details of the wiring and the distribution of neurochemicals, but also by an equally dramatic cultural and intellectual evolution. At the bottom of the lineage, we find clunky stone tools; at today's "top" there are skyscrapers, computers, and biotechnology. Other spinoffs of *Homo*'s evolved brain include language, religion, art, and writing. Simply put, the evolutionary package of neurological changes in *Homo* was unprecedented in the evolutionary histories of other mammals, even including earlier hominids.

I once saw Rudolph Nureyev dance. The steps he did were known to any skilled ballet dancer, but the whole performance clicked in a way I had not seen before. The timing was perfect and the choreography seemed inspired. It was breathtaking. As is true for dance, it is the overall choreography of brain evolution that is unique, not its individual parts or steps. This is why the human brain has failed to evolve new gross structures that differ from those found in the chimpanzee brain.

In conventional dance, such as tap dancing, a shift in the emphasis within certain combinations of steps completely changes the feel of a routine. Thus, the sequence of steps may be identical for two routines, but because of different emphases, the resulting dances are not the same. As evolution progressed, shifts occurred in the timing of developmental events within different parts of *Homo*'s brain. As with dance, change the timing and the resulting brain is not the same. For example, the branching of nerves appears more complex in Broca's speech area on the left side of the human frontal lobe than in the equivalent region on the right. This asymmetry seems to occur because, postnatally, the region on the left develops at a slower rate and for a longer duration than its counterpart on the right. Presumably, this shift in development between right and left hemispheres occurred in conjunction with natural selection for language.

The right hemisphere matures more rapidly than the left during prenatal development as well. Even the slightest shift in the relative maturation rates of the two hemispheres can alter the balance between the specific prenatal hormonal environment and the relative stages of development of the two growing hemispheres. Since hormonal influences differ depending on the stage of development, subtle shifts in maturation rates of the two hemispheres may have provided an underlying mechanism for increased brain lateralization in *Homo*. As others have suggested, prenatal shifts in developmental events may sometimes mark a fine line between mental retardation and giftedness. For the reasons listed above, and because the human brain has yielded numerous aesthetic achievements (such as Nureyev's dance), I refer to *Homo*'s evolutionary trajectory during the past two million years as the braindance.

I believe that Einstein's theory of relativity, Mozart's horn concertos, and the enormous brain of *Homo sapiens* are all due to a fortunate set of serendipitous coincidences that led to this braindance. As discussed in the radiator theory, one coincidence is that some of the protohominids who were preadapted for bipedalism happened to live in just the right thermal environment for achieving both full bipedalism and a big brain. Another happy accident is that these hominids had an impetus for refining their bipedalism because they had to travel to find their daily food and water. By shaping motor patterns, communication skills, and the cleverness needed to survive in such a harsh savanna habitat, natural selection sculpted a subtly rewired human brain.

There is, alas, a dark side to the braindance. As in chimpanzees' brains, the deep part of the human brain that processes emotions (known as the limbic system) causes humans to divide the world into friends and enemies. Consequently people, like chimpanzees, are capable of carrying out atrocious acts of violence against their own kind. The same evolved brain that is responsible for human activities, such as writing poetry or composing symphonies, continues to be fascinated with global military endeavors that could put an abrupt end to the braindance. Although the cortical mechanisms for controlling aggression are part of the neurological package that we inherited from our hominid ancestors, our species needs to exercise vigilantly those controls over our natural primate tendency to engage in

potentially catastrophic dominance interactions. Which will ultimately win out—the braindance, or the brainwar? The choice
is ours.

I am sometimes asked why, given the politics of paleoanthropology, I continue to pursue research on human brain evolution.
The answer is that the long-established tradition of selective interpretation and advocacy in hominid paleontology—and in
other fields where politics comes into play as well—is slowly
being replaced by a new spirit of scientific objectivity. As much
as anything, this book celebrates the investigators whose work is
changing our views of human evolution.

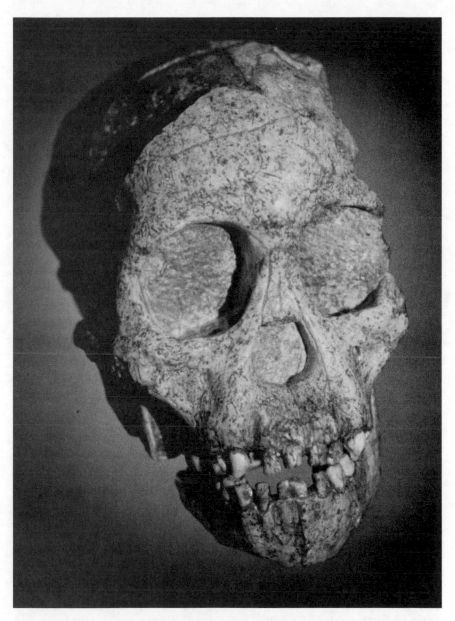

The first australopithecine discovered from Taung, South Africa, in 1924. Known as the Taung "child," this fossil displays a combination of apelike and humanlike features, mostly the former, that had never been seen in living or fossil species before Raymond Dart's discovery. (Photograph by John Reader, copyright © 1992/Science Photo Library)

Clearly, Dart had found a missing link, and he said so in a landmark paper in the February 7, 1925, issue of *Nature*. In that paper, Dart named a new genus and species to accommodate his find; instead of being assigned to *Homo sapiens*, Taung was designated *Australopithecus africanus* ("southern man-ape from Africa"). In keeping with Dart's terminology, the common term used today for Taung and the other earliest known relatives of humans is "australopithecine."

From the outset, Dart and his colleagues overemphasized and overinterpreted the humanlike features of Taung and all other australopithecine fossils. This bias is reflected in Dart's reference to Taung as a "man-ape" instead of an "ape-man" in the title of his 1925 paper.[3] Hindsight suggests two reasons why Dart may have overstated the humanness of australopithecines. The first is historical and should perhaps be viewed with some sympathy. Although Dart knew that Taung "was one of the most significant finds ever made in the history of anthropology" and was sure that Taung was truly a missing link, how was he to persuade the world of this in the anti-intellectual climate that prevailed then? His dilemma becomes apparent when one remembers that less than five months after the announcement of Taung's discovery in *Nature*, John Scopes would be convicted for teaching evolutionary theory to high school students in Dayton, Tennessee (July 21, 1925). At the time the public did not take kindly to the notion of human ancestors as ape-men. Clearly, the more humanlike it was described to be, the more palatable Taung would be as an early hominid ancestor. As mentioned in the Introduction, this situation may have subsequently influenced Dart's assessment of Taung.

The second reason Taung's humanlike features were overemphasized may have been because it was a child. Like humans, other primates go through stages as they grow up. In his analysis of Taung, Dart did not fully appreciate that infant apes have not had time to develop features of the skull, such as thickened eyebrow ridges or attachment areas for heavy neck muscles, that set adult apes apart from humans. Apparently he did not carefully consider the possibility that Taung's rounded forehead or the inferred position of the spinal cord might be due to the immaturity of the apelike specimen rather than to its resemblance to humans.

These observations, made with the advantage of hindsight, are not meant to detract from the fact that Dart made a major contribution to the study of human evolution. Dart lived to be ninety-five years old and had the pleasure of seeing the essence, if not all the details, of his views vindicated. In a field fraught with contention, everyone now agrees that Dart was right about certain things: australopithecines were our earliest known ancestors, they walked on two legs (although not for the reasons Dart believed), and they manifested a combination of apelike and humanlike features. Even Dart's species designation of *Australopithecus africanus* has survived in a discipline that often sinks names shortly after they are proposed.

Much of the foregoing can be found in any introductory textbook on physical anthropology. But the story of the Taung specimen is really more complex. Fossils representing at least thirty australopithecine individuals were found during the 1930s and 1940s. Dart, along with his supporters, again emphasized the humanlike features and downplayed the apelike features of these specimens, possibly in response to early critics who dismissed the importance of these finds. Particularly vexing to these workers was the fact that the brain of Taung was about the size of that of a chimpanzee. In his 1925 article, Dart had claimed that the brain of Taung was humanlike. As it turned out, he was wrong about that.

Dart's biased analysis of Taung began what would become a long tradition of selective interpretation of evidence in paleoanthropology. Today, some workers still promote Dart's view of our earliest ancestors as humanlike because of the australopithecines' bipedalism (Owen Lovejoy of Kent State University), dentition (Alan Mann of University of Pennsylvania), or brain organization (Ralph Holloway of Columbia University). However, these previously accepted conclusions are rapidly being modified as new investigators bring more advanced techniques to the study of hominid evolution. Brigitte Senut (currently of the Musée Nationale d'Histoire Naturelle, Paris) was one of the first to challenge the traditional view, in her 1978 dissertation at the University of Paris, when she showed that the arm bones of certain australopithecines indicated that these bipeds continued to spend a good deal of time in the trees. Based on rigorous analyses of limb bones and joint surfaces, Bill Jungers and his colleagues from the State University of New York at Stony Brook have also argued convincingly that bipedalism in early hominids was not as refined as it is in modern humans. Recent studies of dentition by Holly Smith (University of Michigan) and Tim Bromage (Hunter College) show that the age of death for Taung is better estimated by using information about tooth development for apes than for humans. Furthermore, Glenn Conroy and Michael Vannier (Washington University School of Medicine) have verified this conclusion by using high-resolution computerized tomography (CT scans) to see previously hidden structures in the Taung skull. It now appears that Taung was even younger than initially believed—between three and four years of age, rather than between five and six, as Dart believed.

As Holly Smith points out, an important implication of the finding that the Taung fossil and other early hominids are more apelike than humanlike is that australopithecines matured quickly, as apes do. Based on incremental growth markings in teeth, A. D. Beynon (The Dental School at Newcastle-upon-Tyne) and Christopher Dean (University College, London) concur that, unlike human children, australopithecines did not have prolonged childhoods during which they were educated and socialized by their parents. It is amazing that it has taken nearly sixty-five years to realize these and other important facts about what may be the world's most famous fossil. I attribute these belated realizations to a field that sometimes venerates its established authorities more than it does scientific objectivity. Because of this, the scientific method was slow to arrive at paleoanthropology's doorstep. I can't help but wonder if it wouldn't have gotten there sooner if Josephine Salmons had been invited to dinner in another decade, or if the first australopithecine described had been an adult.

Two Types of Early Hominids:
Australopithecus Big, *Australopithecus* Little

In retrospect, it is curious that it took over ten years for scientists to find adult australopithecines that might have been Taung's "parents." That task fell primarily to Robert Broom, a Scottish physician who had a consuming interest in fossils and was one of the first to recognize the validity of Dart's claim that Taung was a missing link. Today, Broom's picture appears in many textbooks, and appropriately so, for it was he who discovered the very important fact that there was more than one kind of australopithecine.

Broom's first discovery occurred in 1936, when the manager of a lime quarry at Sterkfontein showed him an endocast from an adult hominid. Broom soon found parts of the skull from the same young adult male. Broom was a "splitter"—that is, he tended to give each new fossil a new species name, and that's what he did in this case. Today, however, Broom's first discovery is recognized as a member of the species named by Dart in 1925, *Australopithecus africanus*. Because their skulls are generally more graceful looking than those of the second type of australopithecine (which Broom would not discover for another two years), these hominids are referred to as gracile australopithecines. (Technically, the term hominid refers to members of the family that includes both australopithecines and *Homo*.)

The early history of hominid paleontology is wonderfully romantic. In his book *Finding the Missing Link*, Broom tells how, in 1938, a schoolboy named Gert Terblanche "drew from the pocket of his trousers four of the most wonderful teeth ever seen in the world's history." After Gert showed Broom a site called Kromdraai where he had discovered the teeth, they found and pieced together more of the fossil. When they finished, Broom saw that they had assembled the skull of an adult male australopithecine. However, this one differed from the one found two years earlier at Sterkfontein because it was much more heavily

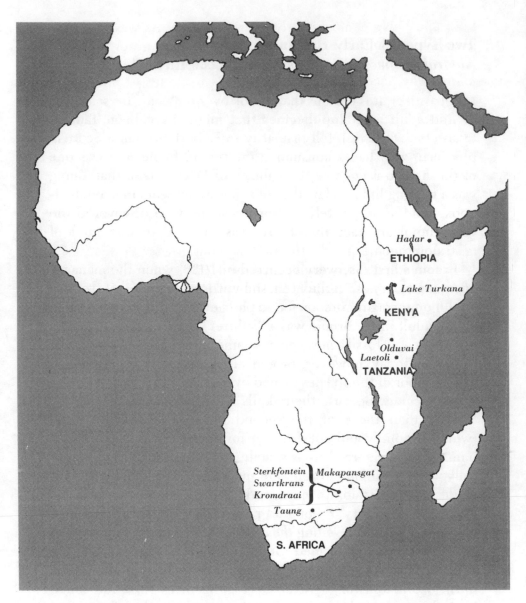

Map of Africa showing the approximate locations of important early hominid discoveries.

while robust australopithecines specialized in a limited menu, gracile australopithecines ate what they could get.

And getting food could be difficult for gracile australopithecines, who, according to Robinson, were dealing "with the stresses of a somewhat hostile environment."[4] Nevertheless, Robinson conceded, "implements for digging will have made possible greater exploitation of . . . bulbs. . . . Implements for bashing, hitting, or throwing . . . will have made capture and consumption of small animals much easier. Improved tool-using will thus have been favored . . ." Clearly, Robinson thought that *Australopithecus* walked on two legs and carried a big stick, and that meat-eating was crucial for the evolution of this early hominid. Although *Paranthropus* probably used tools, wrote Robinson, the "activity may have been much more poorly developed in this vegetarian . . ." And, since tool-using was at a premium among gracile australopithecines, so too was improved intelligence. In short, Robinson thought that gracile australopithecines were less primitive and smarter than robust australopithecines and that they alone gave rise to *Homo*.

On the floor of the hominid vault of the Transvaal Museum in Pretoria, South Africa, there is a narrow open box that contains what appear to be ordinary rocks. Careful scrutiny, however, shows that the rocks have been modified by early hominids. These rocks are therefore known as pebble tools, or Olduwan pebble tools, in honor of Olduvai Gorge, where such artifacts were first recognized. The oldest pebble tools yet discovered are around 2.5 million years old. Ideally, one would like to find a pebble tool held in the hand bones of a complete early hominid skeleton. That hasn't happened yet and, at the moment, we cannot be sure if early stone tools were made by gracile australopithecines, robust australopithecines, or both.

Over fifty years have passed since the discovery of robust australopithecines, and Robinson's early ideas about the relationship between the two types of australopithecines sparkle in comparison with those of many recent workers. Sadly, a recently discovered robust australopithecine skull from Kenya (WT 17000, the Black Skull) has caused current workers to become "splitters" again, i.e., to recognize more rather than fewer species of fossil hominids. (Such efforts may be motivated by attempts to preserve as much as possible of previously published family trees.) Unnecessary splitting serves only to confuse our understanding of the past. On the other hand, Robinson's consolidation of early hominids into two groups and his determination to understand the differences between those two groups *in functional terms* stand as eloquent examples of how to do good science.

It is enthralling to contemplate Dart's discovery of the Taung fossil, about which he wrote "No diamond cutter ever worked more lovingly or with such care on a priceless jewel," or to imagine Broom, the avid collector of scientific specimens, as described in his biography:

> During the collecting campaign Mary Broom, always a self-effacing lady, had to drive in the back-seat of the car next to a recently collected polecat . . . and Broom in front. Says Mary Broom: "Robert, the wee beastie is smelling." Broom: "Impossible! It's still alive."[5]

Robinson's ideas about gracile and robust australopithecines were more than enthralling; they were visionary.

There is a delicious irony associated with the fact that Taung was the type specimen designated by Dart in conjunction with establishing *Australopithecus africanus*. (The type specimen is the ideal against which all other candidates for this taxon are compared.) As noted above, ape and human youngsters go through different stages as they are growing up. It is hard enough to decipher trends in the evolution of adult hominids from those bits of bones and teeth that happen to arrive at museums as fossils, but it is nearly impossible to learn much from those same fossils about the growth of the children of our earliest ancestors. And Taung was a child—a young child. Because of this, we cannot really be sure whether Taung was a gracile or a robust australopithecine.

In 1976, Phillip Tobias suggested that Taung might be a juvenile robust australopithecine, instead of a juvenile gracile australopithecine. That suggestion fell on deaf ears. Since then, several robustlike features have been described in the Taung specimen. These features include the structure of the sinuses in the face and features related to the brain's blood flow. Wouldn't it be ironic if the type specimen for gracile australopithecines turned out really to be a robust australopithecine?

In conclusion, the anti-intellectual climate of the 1920s and the fact that the first australopithecine discovered happened to be a child probably contributed to Dart's incorrect interpretation of australopithecines as more humanlike than apelike. Unfortunately, Dart's biased analysis of Taung established a long tradition of selective interpretation of the hominid fossil record. Today, when new fossil hominids are discovered, there are still some paleoanthropologists who would rather add extraneous branches to their previously published family trees than switch to simpler and more logical branching patterns. When it comes to australopithecines, hominid paleontologists seem to agree on only one point: they came in two basic forms—robust and gracile.

Putting Flesh on the Bones

So fossilized teeth and bones tell us that there were two types of australopithecines. That is all fine and good, but the next important issue is how these early hominids lived. How did they get along with each other? And how are they related to us? Although some guesswork is required to put flesh on australopithecine bones, our ideas about the lives of early hominids are not based on mere speculation. Instead, paleontologists look to living primates for good guesses about how our earliest ancestors behaved.

The two great apes who live in Africa today—the chimpanzee and the gorilla—are genetically close to us, and it is therefore instructive for us to study their distinctive life-styles when attempting to reconstruct the behavior of early hominids. Actually, because the chimpanzee shares a more recent common ancestor with humans than the gorilla does, it is believed to be our closest nonhuman cousin. Like the gracile and robust ape-men, chimpanzees and gorillas live in different environments (environmental niches) and therefore have different life-styles.

Take the Eastern highland gorilla. This largest of living primates has been terribly misunderstood. The Hollywood notion of gorillas as ferocious, charging, chest-beating bullies has been overemphasized. Most of the time, gorillas are peaceful souls. They live in harems ruled by a single confident, dominant silverback male. Although younger blackback males also reside in a harem, it is the silverback who mates with the harem's adult females and consequently fathers all of their infants. His authority is seldom challenged. Younger males eventually leave the group and join other bachelors. One day they may woo females away from other harems (*then* there might be a little chest beating), settle down, and start their own harems. Nevertheless, harems are not generally hostile to each other. And they do not normally compete for food or females.

Life in a gorilla harem is not nearly as sexy as it sounds. In fact, it's relatively boring compared with the more lively goings-on of promiscuous chimpanzees. Gorilla watchers describe the harem as a relatively stable social unit in which sexual encounters are predictable, dull, and infrequent. In keeping with this, the sexual swellings that advertise receptivity in females are not as pronounced as those of the more sexually active chimpanzees. Staid gorillas also engage in little mutual grooming or touching. (Chimpanzees are much more "touchy-feely.")

The day-to-day life of a gorilla seems rather placid. Sunbathing is a favorite pastime. So is eating. Gorillas spend up to eight hours a day consuming tough vegetation, such as bamboo, vines, stalks, bark, roots, and other high-cellulose food. The bulky vegetarian diet of gorillas is reflected in the size of their skulls and teeth. Large canines are used to strip vegetation; and huge chewing muscles are anchored to an enormous face and to the bony crest that runs along the middle of the skull. Oddly enough, the vegetarian diet of gorillas may help explain their harem social life!

Harem organizations are rare among ground-dwelling, Old World primates. Patas monkeys, hamadryas baboons, and gelada baboons live in harems. In each case, associating in small harems instead of larger mixed or multimale groups appears to be a way of coping with food limitations imposed by harsh or uneven environments. Gorillas are strict vegetarians who live in pockets of tropical rain forests. Consequently, their food is dispersed in relatively small patches and it simply will not stretch to feed larger groups.

Because they are so big, adult gorillas spend a good deal of time moving on all fours on the ground (they are terrestrial). They share with chimpanzees a peculiar way of moving across the ground (called knuckle-walking), in which the hands are folded so that the weight of the body is distributed across the knuckles. The shoulders of gorillas are built for climbing and moving in trees, however, and this activity is frequently enjoyed by the lighter weight infants and females. Males are much, much larger than females. Such sexual dimorphism (markedly different appearance of males and females) is associated with male defense of the group (if pressed, a male gorilla *will* defend his harem) and is the norm for ground-living primates in general.

Compared with gorillas, chimpanzees live in the fast lane. They inhabit more varied and dangerous grassland and (in some cases) forest woodland areas. And they eat a wide variety of foods, including vegetables, fruits, nuts, insects, and even meat. Since these foods are not scarce or limited to small pockets in the environment, chimpanzees have forsaken the harem way of life for a much looser form of raucous group living. Their so-called "fusion-fission" society is completely open, and adults of both sexes come and go as they wish.

Promiscuous mating behavior is the norm among chimpanzees. When females become sexually receptive, they enter a hormonal state known as estrus. The genitals of estrous females become very swollen (much more so than those of less adventuresome gorilla females), and this condition is a powerful mating stimulus for both sexes. An estrous chimpanzee may mate with a series of males on one day, and go off to be alone with one particular male on another. Paternity is therefore difficult to determine for chimpanzees.

Although males are somewhat larger than females, sex differ-

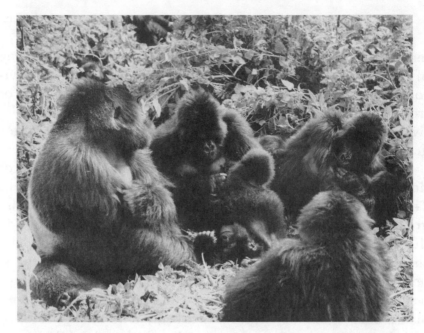

The chimpanzees from Gombe live in the fast lane. Unprotected by mountains or tropical forests, they inhabit the more varied and dangerous lowland grasslands and woodlands. (Photographs courtesy A. H. Harcourt/Anthro-Photo, above, and Curt Busse, below.)

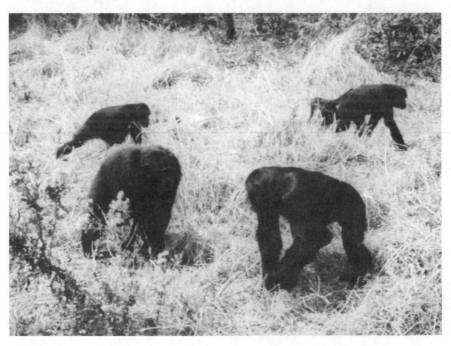

ences in body sizes of chimpanzees are not as marked as those seen in harem primates. Further, the extraordinary large faces and crests of bones associated with chewing muscles in strictly vegetarian gorillas are greatly reduced or missing in the more omnivorous chimpanzees. Chimpanzees are just plain smaller than gorillas.

But what most endears chimpanzees to us are their similarities to humans. They are outgoing and expressive in their social interactions. They greet each other with hugs, kisses, and joyful vocalizations. They like to touch and to clean each other's coats. Chimpanzees are affectionate and imitative in their interactions with humans; their body language is very much like our own.

As Jane Goodall has documented at the Gombe National Park in Tanzania, chimps are also clever. In the wild, they make tools to fish for insects, collect drinking water, and (in the rain forest of the Ivory Coast) crack nuts. Chimpanzees also recognize themselves in mirrors. This has been demonstrated by my colleague at the State University of New York in Albany, Gordon Gallup, who believes that chimpanzees are self-aware and have a sense of "I," much as humans do. Finally, our closest cousins have a certain appeal even in their looks—with big, humanlike ears and frequent premature baldness.

Thanks to Jane Goodall's monumental work, we now know that there is also a darker side to chimpanzee nature. I believe that understanding the Mr. Hyde in chimpanzees is very important for understanding human origins. Unlike gorillas, chimpanzee males form groups to patrol the boundaries of their territory. Groups of males also hunt and eat small mammals, including monkeys and an occasional chimpanzee infant. And these activities are undertaken with a bloodlust that is rarely seen in other primates—except for *Homo sapiens* (but more about that later).

From Apes to Ape-men

The fieldwork that has been carried out on certain groups of chimpanzees and gorillas provides clues about how the two types of australopithecines may have lived: it is possible that robust australopithecines occupied a niche that in some ways resembled that of living highland gorillas. Gracile australopithecines, on the other hand, may have had a life-style more like that of the grassland and woodland chimpanzees from Gombe. It is important to note, however, that the similarities between ape-men and apes would have been channeled by environmental variables such as availability of preferred food, and not by the existence of different apelike ancestors for the two kinds of hominid. Indeed, both on molecular and fossil evidence, paleontologists firmly believe that both types of australopithecines shared one apelike common ancestor.

What evidence is there for this? Recall that the two ape-men are physically distinct in the dental and facial features because of their different diets. Paleontologists agree that robust australopithecines were strict vegetarians who specialized in hard foods; gracile australopithecines were not. This alone shows that the two ape-men occupied distinct niches. But what is there to suggest that robust australopithecines behaved like gorillas? Or that gracile hominids acted more like grassland and woodland chimpanzees?

Robust australopithecines probably lived in cooler forested habitats, more in keeping with those occupied today by gorillas than by the Gombe chimpanzees. All robust australopithecines have a circulatory system for the brain that is associated with living in cooler rather than hotter habitats. Furthermore, the finger and toe bones of the probable ancestors of robust australopithecines are curved. This indicates that these hominids, although basically bipedal, nevertheless retained the general apelike habit of spending some time in trees (and therefore in treed habitats). Like gorillas, robust australopithecines are characterized by marked sexual dimorphism. And, of course, like gorillas, the diet of robust australopithecines was extremely specialized and strictly vegetarian. (It is important to note, however, that the teeth of australopithecines differ in various ways from those of apes.)

But can we infer anything about the actual behavior of robust australopithecines? We probably can. The combination of strict vegetarian diet, marked sexual dimorphism, and basic ground-living suggests that these early hominids lived in harems.[6] As with contemporary harem primates, males probably defended their harems as was necessary. However, interharem relationships would have been primarily peaceful, with harems joining to form larger groups for defense—as food and circumstances warranted.

That is not to say that robust australopithecines were *exactly* like gorillas. Although males were markedly larger than females, very recent findings suggest that neither sex of robust hominids may have been so robust after all![7] Robustness may have been confined to structures related to chewing, while the rest of the body remained relatively slight. This is obviously not the case for gorillas. Nor are gorillas known for tool use, or for being particularly intelligent. However, the degree to which robust australopithecines used tools, as well as the extent of their general intelligence, are questions that remain tantalizingly open.[8]

And what about gracile australopithecines? Is there evidence to suggest that they lived more like grassland and woodland chimpanzees than like gorillas? As a matter of fact, there is. Several recent workers have seconded Robinson's belief that gracile australopithecines lived in open savanna grasslands and therefore were subject to more solar radiation than their forest-dwelling cousins. This suggestion receives support from fossilized scraps of gracile australopithecines from Laetoli, Tanzania, that are about 3.5 million years old. One specimen, a portion of the skull, shows that these early hominids did *not* have the kind of circulatory system for the brain that seems to be associated with cooler habitats and is found in all robust australopithecines. Moreover, the famous footprints that Mary Leakey discovered at Laetoli appear to have been made by feet that lacked the curved tree-clinging toes of robust australopithecines. It seems, indeed, that gracile australopithecines were out in the open. Out in the open and getting hot in the sun. (Later it will be shown that this has important consequences for how brain temperature is regulated.)

Male and female gracile australopithecines may not have differed as dramatically in their body sizes as robust australopithecines did. And their teeth tell us that they ate softer fruits and foliage than did their robust cousins. The combination of these features, along with woodland or savanna living, are found in the chimpanzees from Gombe and seem to go with a multimale social organization. Gracile australopithecines may also have lived in promiscuous, open groups. They may have had a taste for meat, which they would satisfy, catch-as-catch-can, by various means, including scavenging the kills of other animals. I also think they had a taste for salt.

So much for speculation about the day-to-day lives of gracile and robust australopithecines. What we would really like to know is what they were like cognitively. And how intelligent they were. Although this may sound like an impossible goal, South Africa has produced a dazzling record of australopithecine natural endocasts that have revealed details about the cerebral cortex of our earliest hominid ancestors. I have been very fortunate to be involved in the investigation of these and other hominid fossils. My research, which can best be described as stormy, began fourteen years ago in a room known as the Red Cave.

Into the Cave

In the basement of the Transvaal Museum in Pretoria, South Africa, there is an exceedingly thick bank-vault door. Behind this door is the Red Cave—a small room that contains a priceless collection of fossils from our earliest ape-men ancestors. I first visited the Transvaal Museum during the summer of 1978 to study the more humdrum fossils of monkeys. Each time I passed by the locked vault, I longed to enter the Red Cave. As a newcomer to the museum, however, I knew my wish to study these glamorous fossils of our earliest ancestors was too much to hope for. After all, from my recent graduate-school perspective, the field of hominid paleontology seemed dominated by just a few privileged workers and this inner circle was notorious for being difficult to

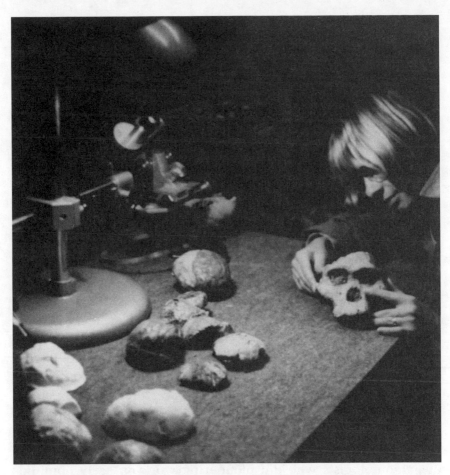

The author studies the braincase of Mrs. Ples in the Red Cave, 1978; other natural hominid endocasts await inspection on the table.

penetrate.[9] I kept to my monkey fossils. And the door to the hominid vault remained closed.

Near the end of my stay in Pretoria, I decided to examine some unidentified fossils that were kept in boxes in an out-of-the-way storage room. In one dusty, forgotten box marked "unidentified monkeys," I found a small fossil that was *not* monkey. It was hominid! But would I be able to convince museum officials that it was? I spent two days poring over reference books and monkey fossils in order to prepare my case. Carefully, I arranged the specimen, numerous illustrations, and some monkey fossils on a table. After rehearsing my arguments several times, I was ready. I sought out the director of the museum, Bob Brain, and asked somewhat hesitantly, "Excuse me, Dr. Brain. I wonder if I could show you something for a moment?"

"Why of course, Dean," he said, accompanying me to my display. As he looked at the specimen, I took a deep breath in preparation for my arduous explanation. Before I could say one word, Dr. Brain said with obvious delight, "Why, you've found a hominid, haven't you!" Subsequently, Brain and another official at the museum, Elisabeth Vrba (now at Yale), encouraged me to compare the fossil with the other hominids and to publish my findings. So the door to the Red Cave was opened to me after all. When I first entered that room, I had no idea of the secrets it would reveal.

The hominid vault at the Transvaal Museum is the most amazing room I've ever been in. It is small, rectangular, and the color scheme is blood red. (Vrba selected the color; she said it was that or purple.) The walls are lined with antique glass cabinets containing red velvet boxes—boxes that hold treasures. Imagine entering this room and finding yourself face-to-face (so to speak) with an array of fossil skulls (such as the gracile australopithecine nicknamed "Mrs. Ples" and the original robust *Paranthropus*) that are pictured in most paleoanthropology textbooks! Photographs of paleontologists who did pioneering work on early hominids decorate the walls and there is a small worktable. Someone on the staff brings a space heater (it's winter there in June); then you are left to ponder the fossils. Your only interruption is the sound of a bell tinkling as an employee walks through the museum calling the staff to tea.[10]

Ever since I was rescued from undergraduate doldrums by an inspiring teacher, Charles Reed, I have been interested in the evolution of the human brain. Thanks to Charles, a zoologist (and one of those rare scholar/teachers), my initial interest was in the volume of the braincase, a feature known as cranial capacity and measured in cubic centimeters (cm^3). Cranial capacities of our ancestors reveal a startling fact. Brain size in living humans is almost four times as large as it was in our hominid relatives who lived over three million years ago. Even when we consider that

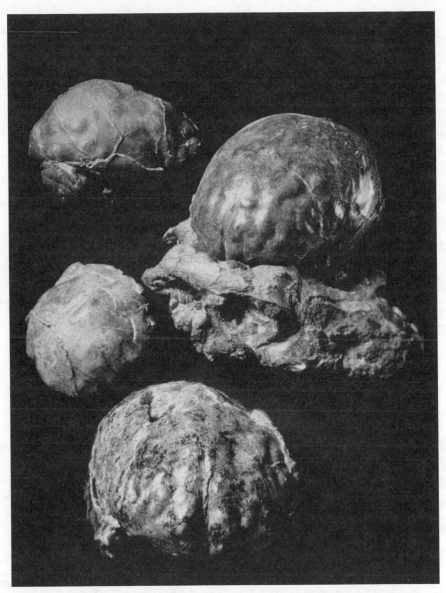

The natural endocasts of South African australopithecines. Early hominid skulls filled up with fine, lime-rich sediments that then became fossilized. Each endocast preserves in unusual detail the external brain convolutions and blood vessels that left their imprint inside the cranium. (Photograph by John Reader, copyright © 1992/ Science Photo Library)

body size has also increased dramatically, this increase in brain size is unprecedented in mammals. Nothing like it has been seen before. Why did the brains of our ancestors enlarge as they did? When I first stepped into the Red Cave, I had no idea. Fourteen years later, I have an inkling—and it's presented in this book.

The little fossil that I disinterred from the dusty box was not part of the skull or, for that matter, any other part of the skeleton. What I had found was a cast of the interior of the braincase of an individual who had lived between 2.5 and 3 million years ago. Like the Taung endocast, this naturally occurring endocast revealed details of the brain that had been imprinted on the inside of the braincase. Although endocasts may be prepared artificially from skulls (using latex), the occurrence of natural endocasts is a rare event that depends on highly favorable geological conditions. Unfortunately for paleontologists, these conditions exist in few places in the world. South Africa is one. The result is a remarkable record of natural endocasts for the animals that lived there, and it is fortunate that our earliest ancestors were among those who unwittingly took advantage of this geological opportunity. What beginner's luck I had in finding one of these hominid endocasts (only the seventh ever found) while rummaging in a museum box.

For all practical purposes, I carried in my hand a small portion of the cerebral cortex of an ape-man when I first entered the Red Cave. Imagine the feeling! Six other hominid natural endocasts awaited inspection, and they were more complete than the little specimen I had found. (The Taung specimen, arguably the most important early hominid endocast, was located in the Department of Anatomy at the University of Witwatersrand in Johannesburg, rather than in the Red Cave. The head of that department, Professor Phillip Tobias, kindly allowed me to study that specimen.) Although brain size in these early hominids was as small as that of chimpanzees, Dart's notion that australopithecine endocasts looked like miniature versions of modern human brains had nearly achieved the status of a received truth by the time I set foot in the Red Cave. Indeed, no other view existed in the contemporary paleontological literature. That is why, in

1978, I fully expected to see humanlike sulcal patterns on early hominid endocasts. However, as I examined the hominid endocasts, I found, to my astonishment, that this was not the case. The folds of gray matter reproduced on the endocasts were *not* humanlike. Instead, they appeared completely apelike. At least to me they did.

The Beginnings of Controversy

In 1979, the late Leonard Radinsky published observations questioning the humanlike affinities of the Taung endocast. I followed suit in 1980 and published findings that all seven early hominid natural endocasts (including Taung) appeared apelike rather than humanlike. After all, the early hominids of South Africa had brains that were roughly the size of those of chimpanzees. So it should not have been surprising to find that the pattern of convolutions on the Red Cave endocasts appeared similar to those on chimpanzee brains. Right? Wrong. It amuses me now to recall my belief that findings that flew in the face of conventional wisdom would be accepted by the field, as long as the supporting evidence from chimpanzee, gorilla, and human brains was published with the conclusions.

In my 1980 paper, I unwittingly reopened a controversy that had lain dormant for fifty-five years by pointing out that when Dart first described the Taung endocast, he mistook the lambdoid suture of the skull for the lunate sulcus of the brain. The lambdoid suture is an irregular edge on the skull that is formed by the fusion of the occipital and parietal bones. A sulcus is a narrow valley that separates convolutions of the brain, and the lunate sulcus is a crescent-shaped groove (hence its name) that is located at the front end of the occipital lobe, which processes visual information in monkeys, apes, and humans. However, when one compares brains representing these three groups of primates, one discovers that the lunate sulcus is located *much farther back in the human brain* than on the others. Because he misidentified the lambdoid suture as the lunate sulcus, Dart claimed that the lunate sulcus was located in a humanlike position, far back on the Taung endocast. In other words, it was an unfortunate error that caused Dart to suggest that australopithecine brains were humanlike.[11] Oh, the poor beleaguered lunate sulcus! Its significance for hominid brain evolution was doomed to be misunderstood from the word *go*.

If the feature that Dart identified wasn't Taung's lunate sulcus, then where was it? As an alternative, I suggested that a small dimple near the top of the Taung endocast might represent one end of the lunate sulcus. (The whole lunate sulcus did not show up on Taung or on any of the other six australopithecine endocasts.) This dimple was in a relatively forward location that was consistent with an apelike position for the lunate sulcus. To me, such an interpretation seemed logical because of the *overall* apelike sulcal patterns on these specimens. (If the dimple did not represent the end of the lunate sulcus, then any trace of the lunate sulcus simply did not appear on the South African specimens, and nothing more could then be said about that sulcus on these endocasts.)

Ralph Holloway of Columbia University had long championed the Old Guard view that the brains of our earliest ancestors appeared to be humanlike. It is safe to say that he was not happy with my observations. Since my 1980 article on the australopithecine natural endocasts, Holloway and I have engaged in an exchange of fifteen publications that can most kindly be described as lively. That I was able to publish my viewpoint at all in such a contentious field was remarkable and was due in large part to the concern shown by my mentor, Len Radinsky, and his intercession with editors.

The Emperor Has No Clothes!

Politics of the field aside, what were Holloway and I arguing about? Holloway objected to my identification of Taung's dimple as a possible marker for the lunate sulcus. In true the-emperor-has-a-beautiful-suit-of-clothes fashion, Holloway took a new investigator to task for having the nerve to question Dart's authority.[12] According to Holloway,

> it is reasonable to remind readers of this paper of . . . important historical facts: . . . Raymond Dart was a protégé of G. E. Smith, who devoted a very considerable portion of his professional career to the study of the lunate sulcus. Dart's early publications were in comparative neuroanatomy. These points are only mentioned to indicate that those who did study the original specimens were well-versed regarding comparative neuroanatomy, and the lunate sulcus in particular.[13]

Of course, the fact that Smith and Dart were renowned scientists had nothing to do with the actual location of the lunate sulcus on the Taung endocast. Dart had misidentified the lambdoid suture as the lunate sulcus—period. Furthermore, by the time of his 1981 response to my paper, Holloway had quietly shifted away from his 1975 statement that "only a few hominid endocasts [particularly the original Taung (1924) endocast] show the sulcus clearly. . . ."[14] Indeed, Holloway's 1981 view of Taung's lunate sulcus was now that *"we cannot prove where the lunate sulcus is located, but only demonstrate where it is not."*[15]

Would the lunate sulcus finally be allowed to rest in peace? No way. In a series of papers, Holloway continued his offense against Taung's poor little dimple. According to him, my identification was incorrect because the dimple was too far forward to be the lunate sulcus, even of an ape. At times, I just wanted to let the whole thing drop but, prodded and encouraged by my colleagues, I met each offense with a statistical or theoretical defense. Round and round we went. Points of methodology became bones of contention. For example, we debated which methods were better for studying early hominid endocasts: measuring projection and profile indices from photographs or using a stereoplotter to measure details of sulcal patterns. We were getting nowhere slowly (and probably nauseating more than a few readers in the process).

In 1985, I wrote:

I hope that one year from now I will not be writing the seventh paper in this series. Obviously, neither Holloway nor I are changing our opinions about the cortical morphology of australopithecines. . . . It is time that other workers examine the evidence and contribute to this discussion. My laboratory and endocast collection are available to other researchers (or their students) who are interested in this problem.[16]

Unfortunately, there were no takers, and only four years later, in 1989, I found myself publishing the thirteenth article in the lunate sulcus series. (I wanted to entitle it "Lunate Sulcus Paper 13," but the editor would not permit that.) And the subject of this paper? Again, the dimple. Would this controversy ever be put to rest? Would other workers ever stick their necks out and take a position? As it turns out, the answer to both questions was yes.

The problem with the lunate sulcus is that it simply was not reproduced on the South African australopithecine natural endocasts with any clarity. If a clear lunate sulcus had appeared on the Taung or other endocasts, it would have been a good indicator of the extent to which early hominid brains had evolved toward a humanlike condition. A forward position of the lunate sulcus would have suggested an apelike brain. If the lunate sulcus were located in a posterior position, on the other hand, the brain would have appeared humanlike. The dimple on the Taung endocast that I identified as a possible marker for the lunate sulcus was in an apelike position, but Ralph Holloway would have none of that. Since there were no other potential lunate sulci on the South African endocasts, clearly what was needed were other endocasts of early hominids.

In 1985, I had the chance to study the sulcal pattern on another australopithecine endocast, this time from the Hadar formation in Ethiopia (home of Lucy).[17] Dated to about 3.2 million years ago, this specimen (AL 162-28) was older than the South African endocasts. With a cranial capacity of 350–400 cm^3, it was also some 10–20 percent smaller. Most important, the AL 162-28 endocast revealed a beautiful, whole lunate sulcus in addition to numerous other sulci. Like the South African specimens, the entire sulcal pattern of this Hadar endocast was clearly apelike. What was especially frustrating was that when a clear lunate sulcus at last appeared on an australopithecine endocast, Holloway failed to recognize it. Instead, he claimed that for AL 162-28 "there are no landmarks . . . which can be interpreted as a pongid-like lunate sulcus."[18] (Holloway attributed the groove in question to an artifact caused by lipping at the edge of a bone.) In exasperation, I wrote the following poem:

ODE TO THE LUNATE SULCUS

Oh crescent shaped groove near the back of the brain,
Anterior limit of the visual cortex.
So misunderstood, misidentified and misbegotten
In the study of human brain evolution.
In 1925 Dart wrongly identified the lambdoid suture
On the Taung endocast as you!
And others believed it was far back,
So "human, human," they cried,
Although you rarely leave your mark on endocasts,
This does not stop them from guessing your location.
"Human, human," they wail.
And when you finally do reveal yourself,
Splendidly, completely, unequivocally (on AL 162-28),
But, alas, in an apelike position,
"Artifact, artifact," they cry.
Neither calipers, nor stereoplotting, nor projection
Indices have saved you from your fate.
Poor thing.

Although neither calipers, nor stereoplotting, nor projection indices saved the lunate sulcus from its agony, powerful new imaging tools were being developed by Michael Vannier, currently director of the Radiology Research Division at Mallinckrodt Institute of Radiology in St. Louis. These tools would help change Taung's fate.

from rhesus monkey skulls), we would be able to investigate a number of important questions about the neuroanatomy of the most widely used higher primate model in medicine. The extent of cortical asymmetry (or right/left differences) could be explored, and age-related changes in external brain morphology could be quantified. We could also investigate whether or not there were sex differences in the superficial appearance of the brain. Finally, we would be able to do something never before attempted with primates. Because maternal genealogies would be known, we could quantify the contribution of genetic factors (called heritabilities) to variations in the lengths and patterns of brain features.

Mike agreed to participate in the project. Together, we organized a team to carry it out. Over time, the team put together a successful research proposal for funds to support our work.[1] This was our plan: I would make over four hundred endocasts and would collect certain information from them by eyeball. Mike would write the software and direct the collection of data from the endocasts in his laboratory. Charles (Scooter) Hildebolt would draw on the skills he had developed as a dentist in another life (before obtaining a Ph.D. in anthropology) and use his steady hand for the delicate but tedious job of digitizing thousands and thousands of sulci on hundreds and hundreds of endocasts. Finally, Jim Cheverud (a big, brilliant teddy bear) would join our efforts and carry out all of the quantitative and genetic analyses. (Jim was at Northwestern University when the project began and had already done genetic studies on the same skeletons that provided the endocasts. He is now in the Department of Anatomy and Neurobiology at Washington University.) All four of us would participate in the interpretation, writing, and publication of results.

As the project evolved, I periodically flew from Lafayette, Indiana, to St. Louis to meet with the team. Once we got the bugs worked out by doing pilot work, the investigation went remarkably well and, eventually, we obtained exciting results. (Jim made us do lots of pilot work before he was satisfied that we would get meaningful data. However, it was worth it, and we have forgiven

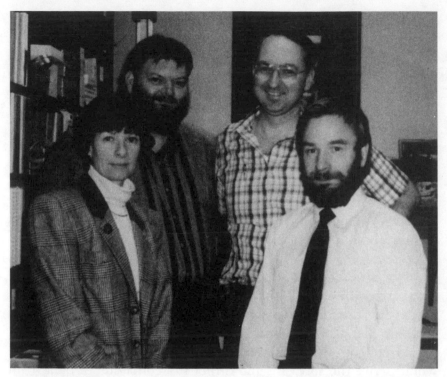

The St. Louis team (left to right): Dean Falk, Jim Cheverud, Mike Vannier, and Charles Hildebolt. A research team that clicked because we responded to each other's exuberance about the work at hand.

him for cracking the whip.) Clearly, we clicked as a team. Looking back on it, I think this happened because all four of us tend toward workaholism, and we, as kindred spirits, responded to each other's exuberance about the work at hand. I grew to love my visits to St. Louis and I still do research there.

Scooter Has an Idea

Scooter usually picks me up at the airport; then we put in a long day at the lab. Frequently, we will use the 3Space to digitize all of the sulci on actual brains. (Scooter digitizes, while I keep a running map of what he is doing.) At other times, we will prepare illustrations or experiment with a new toy that has appeared in the lab since my last visit. Whatever our research agenda, we always find time for idle chitchat. (It amuses me to remember the countless hours we spent discussing whether or not Mike is really an Einstein-caliber genius.)

One day, while we were working with the 3Space, Scooter said to me, "Hey Dean, guess what's in the *American Journal of Physical Anthropology* that just arrived?"

"I give up."

"An article by Ralph Holloway," he said.

"Oh, no," I uttered in dismay. "What's it about?"

"It's another one of those 'apples and oranges' articles," Scooter answered. (He was referring to the title of one of my papers in the exchange with Holloway.)

"Oh, N-o-o-o," I wailed in my "Mr. Bill" voice.

"Dean, don't worry. Nobody actually *reads* those things anymore."

As we continued digitizing, we started talking about the frustrations I had encountered during my long debate with Holloway about australopithecine endocasts. A key problem had to do with the different brain sizes of chimpanzees and humans. Adult human brains are about four times the size of adult chimpanzee brains. Because of the physical laws that govern the relationship between surface areas of brains and their volumes, human brains have more sulci than chimpanzee brains—just because they are bigger. (This is known as allometric scaling.) Before true evolutionary differences can be identified, one must subtract out changes that are due simply to size scaling, or allometry.

In 1980, I had shown that the endocast of Taung had a simpler pattern of convolutions (i.e., fewer sulci) than one would see on a human brain. In fact, the Taung endocast was within the ape range for size and, consistent with this, its sulcal pattern appeared to be apelike rather than humanlike.

"How can I rule out allometric scaling as the only cause for the differences between the Taung endocast and human brains? How can it be shown that Taung's endocast is apelike even after size effects have been subtracted out?" I asked Scooter.

"Digitize the Taung endocast and digitize a human brain that is the same size," Scooter suggested.

"But Scooter, human brains are over three times as big as Taung."

"Not all human brains, Dean."

"What are you talking about, Charles?"

He answered my question with a question, "How old did Taung live to be?"

"Scooter, you know it was a so-called 'baby,' maybe three and a half years old."

"Well, there you go, Dean. Get a brain of a human baby."

The Baby Brain

Of course. A baby brain. Charles's idea was inspired. But finding a normal brain of a human baby was easier said than done. We made requests to various institutions to borrow a baby brain. Very few parents have the altruism and desire to donate their children's bodies to science. When these rare specimens do become available, every effort is made to share them and to maximize the medical, educational, and scientific benefits of these precious gifts to life. Several months after we made our requests, a specimen was loaned to us for our noninvasive research.

It was a beautiful specimen. The brain had been obtained from a two-week-old baby who had died of nonneurological causes. Serendipitously, its volume turned out to be 432 cm^3, so close to the 404 cm^3 estimated for the Taung endocast that it was difficult to tell by eyeball which of the two was bigger. Since human brains have their sulci in place by birth, this would indeed be a good specimen to compare with Taung.

We also intended to compare the baby brain and Taung endocast with the brain of a juvenile chimpanzee that had been part of my scientific collection for many years. It is standard practice for anthropologists to obtain such specimens by requesting that zoos save the carcasses of animals that die from natural causes. As with human specimens, these specimens are highly valued and are frequently shared by a number of investigators.

Departure day for St. Louis. On an earlier trip to South Africa,

Phillip Tobias had given me a copy of the Taung endocast. (Before bringing it home, I compared it feature by feature with the original fossil and found it to be an exquisite copy.) That treasure went into my purse. (I would never check such luggage through in a suitcase.) The chimpanzee brain was in a canister of fluid, which I wrapped in a dark plastic bag and carried by hand. My first plane landed a bit late, and I had to make a very quick connection. Briefcase and purse over my left shoulder, plastic-wrapped container cradled in my right arm, and boarding pass between my teeth—running through the airport. Slosh-slosh-slosh. I was the last person to arrive at the gate.

"Almost didn't make it, huh," the stewardess said in a cheerful manner as she took the boarding pass from my mouth. "What you got there?" she said, eyeing my dark green bundle.

"Uuuhhh," I fumbled as the world went into slow motion and I desperately thought "what'll I tell her? Should I lie? No, she would see right through me—better to tell the truth."

"A chimpanzee brain," I answered feebly.

She paused. "Oohh, a chimpanzee brain," she said in a high, incredulous voice. I held my breath. Then she swept her arm in a wide arc and said "Step right on." We did.

I always find airplane takeoffs exhilarating. This one was particularly so. With Taung in my purse and the chimpanzee brain locked securely between my feet, we were hurtled down the runway. As we ascended, I imagined a little hominid brain being propelled through the millennia and into the Space Age. Taung was on its way to St. Louis.

Taung Meets the 3Space

Scooter digitized; I mapped. Sulcus by sulcus and lobe by lobe. Because the Taung endocast consisted mostly of the right hemisphere, we digitized all of the sulci on the outside surfaces of the right hemisphere of the chimpanzee and baby brains. To check for accuracy, we digitized everything twice. Scooter's years of probing around in people's mouths paid off. His steady hand and the 3Space's ability to measure exact locations proved to be an amazingly accurate partnership. When we were done, we had obtained and stored a voluminous amount of information about the surfaces (or cerebral cortices) of juvenile-chimpanzee and human-baby brains. This would provide the data base for assessing the hominid endocast and would also be saved for future research.

Digitizing the Taung endocast was another matter. Unlike actual brains, endocasts of early hominids pick up only parts of the sulcal pattern. In the case of Taung, fairly good sulcal patterns appear on the right frontal and temporal lobes. (Unfortunately, details are poor on Taung's parietal and occipital lobes.) We digitized all of Taung's visible sulci and, for comparative purposes, also digitized the same set of sulci on the chimpanzee and baby brains. (This was in addition to digitizing the entire surfaces of the two brains, as described above.) Again, everything was done twice and, again, Scooter's steady hand came through. The two sets of measurements of the various sulcal lengths were virtually identical.

Harry Jerison, who is a leading expert on the brain and intelligence and knows as much about allometry as anyone,[2] kindly helped design our quantitative analyses.[3] We used formulas determined from both mammalian data and solid geometry to generate predictions about the expected ratios of sulci on the chimpanzee brain and the Taung endocast, relative to the baby brain. We then compared our predictions with 3Space acquired reality. The results were startling. When brain size was accounted for, the chimpanzee brain had longer (summed) sulci than the endocast of Taung in all areas that could be compared, relative to the human brain. Our results on lengths of sulci confirmed our other observations based on sulcal pattern (in temporal and frontal lobes) and position of the cerebellum. In all respects, the Taung endocast was apelike, not humanlike.

Interestingly, the frontal lobe of Taung turned out to be particularly impoverished in terms of summed sulcal length. The pattern of sulci in the frontal lobe was also extremely simple and

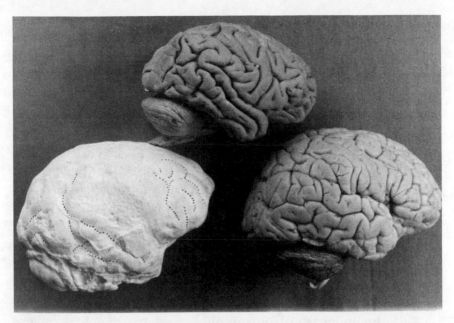

Right hemispheres of a chimpanzee brain (top), the Taung endocast (left), and a human baby brain (right). In all major respects, the Taung endocast appears apelike, not humanlike.

included an orbitofrontal sulcus that is found in ape brains but not in human brains. (This is also true of all scorable australopithecine endocasts.) Este Armstrong, a Distinguished Scientist at the Armed Forces Institute of Pathology, and her colleagues have recently shown that, of all the lobes of the brain, the frontal lobes of humans are the most convoluted compared with those of apes.[4] From Armstrong's work and our own, it appears that frontal lobes became more convoluted relatively recently, i.e., after the divergence of *Homo* from the australopithecines. Thus, the frontal lobes are of key importance for understanding human brain evolution.

It has been a long haul, this research on australopithecine endocasts. Traditionally, paleoanthropologists have emphasized the humanlike attributes of australopithecines and downplayed their apelike features. (After all, these were our relatives.) When I entered the Red Cave, australopithecines were thought to be humanlike in their teeth, limbs, and pelves, as well as in their cortical sulcal patterns. Many researchers also believed that australopithecines were as refined in their bipedalism as contemporary humans.

But, the emperor now has no clothes. Since 1985, much new evidence has come to light that shows australopithecines were much more apelike than previously believed. As I write this book, the accepted view of Taung and the other australopithecines has taken a 180-degree turn because of the research on dentition and locomotion by numerous young investigators whose work has already been discussed: Bill Jungers, Holly Smith, Tim Bromage, Mike Vannier, and Glenn Conroy. Although the "australopithecines-are-humanlike" school still has its diehards, they no longer hold the majority opinion. The voices of the young Turks of paleontology have finally risen above the cacophony of contention.

And, the endocasts of australopithecines are, of course, just as apelike as they can be. Furthermore, as I had hoped would happen, other workers have finally published their views on hominid brain evolution. Recent research by Armstrong and her colleagues (using advanced techniques on different primates) and by Jerison (based on comparative morphometric considerations) supports the contention that the lunate sulcus of early hominids was in an apelike location.[5]

Looking for Mr. Goodbrain

The australopithecine natural endocasts from South Africa have created a dilemma: if the hominids that lived between roughly two and three million years ago appeared to be apelike in their brains, when did a humanlike brain first appear in the fossil record? Moreover, which part of the brain should we look to for an answer to this question? The one area of the cortex that best distinguishes an ape brain from a human brain is the frontal lobes. A triangular fold of gray matter known as Broca's area appears in left frontal lobes of humans and is associated with speech. This area does not appear in ape brains. Not only is the lower frontal lobe the best area for distinguishing an ape brain from a human brain, but it is also the area which is most likely to leave a good impression on the inside of the skull and therefore appear on an endocast—a happy accident.

By 1980, I knew that humanlike brains were not showing up in the fossil record of hominids that lived over two million years ago. It was time to move forward in the fossil record, but that meant gaining access to fossils in other parts of Africa. Because of the dispute with Holloway, my work was already controversial. How would curators react to my request to study their collections? Although I was denied access to some fossils, I believe it was out of a sheer sense of fair play that one museum director let me into the shop. In 1982, I went to the National Museums of Kenya to study the fossil hominids under Richard Leakey's care.

I love to visit Nairobi. It's fast-paced and so African (compared with South Africa which somehow feels more like Europe) with its wonderful sights, smells, and restaurants. I get excited just taking a taxi in from the airport to the Hotel Boulevard (which has supplanted the New Ainsworth Hotel as *the* place for museum visitors to stay). It's right next to the museum on Casino Hill. Moreover, it is reasonably priced, clean, and has passable food. The best thing, however, is that many scientists who visit the museum from June through August stay there, and a wonderful camaraderie develops between these clients of the hotel. It's like being at science camp.

Just up the hill from the hotel is a statue of Louis Leakey. He is perched on a pile of rocks, with a stone tool in his hand. Behind that statue is the National Museums of Kenya. It too has a hominid vault. Although less colorful than the Red Cave, this vault is larger and its fossils are more varied, reflecting the fact that the East African australopithecines were not alone. They had company.

What spectacular hominids there were between one and two million years ago in East Africa. As hard as it is to imagine, the robust australopithecines from East Africa looked even more rugged than those from South Africa (hence they are sometimes described as hyper-robust). As with variations among the human races today, these differences seem to have been associated with living in different regions. The gracile australopithecines in East Africa had somewhat bigger brains than those from South Africa, but this is hardly surprising since they lived more recently.

Simon Kasinga of the National Museums of Kenya and I prepared endocasts from the most complete fossil skulls there. What resulted was confirmation that even these relatively recent robust and gracile australopithecines appeared apelike in their cerebral cortices. Mr. (Ms.) Goodbrain was not to be found among these specimens.

East Africa was a busy place one to two million years ago. It was there and at that time that another group of hominids was undergoing extremely rapid evolution. I refer of course to our own genus, *Homo*. The oldest known species in this lineage is *Homo habilis,* who at some undetermined point in time branched off from gracile australopithecine stock. Most paleoanthropologists agree that *Homo habilis* gave rise to *Homo erectus,* who in turn gave rise to *Homo sapiens.* The transition between *Homo habilis* and *Homo erectus* seems to have occurred rapidly and exclusively in Africa.[6]

Brain size increased with incredible swiftness in the genus *Homo*. But what concerns us here is the surface structure of the cerebral cortex. During the summer of 1982, Simon Kasinga and I cast the braincase of the oldest skull representing *Homo habilis*. And guess what. Unlike any of the australopithecine endocasts, this one (from specimen KNM-ER 1470) appeared to be humanlike in the revealing convolutions of its left frontal lobe. As Phillip Tobias first suggested, *Homo habilis* appears to have had a Broca's speech area in its brain and, as such, was probably capable of some form of rudimentary humanlike language.

Our lineage has evolved dramatically since the first glimmerings of language appeared in the brain of *Homo habilis.* As brain size rapidly doubled, its plethora of connections became increasingly complex. The overall floorplan of the cerebral cortex also changed. The cultural products of the cerebral cortex evolved too. Over time, transportation developed from unshod feet to airplanes. The spoken word gave rise to writing and numbers—to information technology that in turn has led to the computer revolution and, now, the dawning of biotechnology. Our ancestors' ability to conceive of making a few clunky stone tools occurred at the beginning of a neurological trajectory that would one day result in Mozart's horn concertos and Einstein's theory of relativity. As we shall see, all of this was heralded in the endocast of ER 1470. Two million years ago, the braindance had begun.

But I am getting ahead of myself. How can we assess the importance of the different appearances of australopithecine and *Homo* endocasts without understanding something about the differences between ape and human brains and what these differences mean for cognition?

Kanzi?" Surprisingly, although Kanzi communicates mainly through gestures and pressing keyboard symbols, he also attempts to say the following English words/phrases: "carrot," "onion," "raisin," "snake," "right now," and "open"!

As with young humans, Kanzi's language comprehension is ahead of his language production. Most of his utterances are one or two words. His linguistic skills continue to increase as he matures, although not as much as those of a human child. Kanzi is not alone. The Language Research Center houses three other bonobos, five common chimpanzees, and two orangutans, all of whom participate in language studies. The findings for Kanzi have been confirmed: young apes, like young children, can assimilate certain language skills by observing and listening to their caretakers.

But there are certain language-related skills that apes, even young apes, do *not* develop. Savage-Rumbaugh points out that whereas humans can do simultaneous tasks, chimpanzees cannot. (In other words, chimps have a hard time with the proverbial problem of walking and chewing gum at the same time.) Savage-Rumbaugh also notes that chimpanzees can invent gestures fairly easily, but these inventions do not get encoded and transmitted to others. This may be due to the fact that chimpanzees have difficulty cooperating with each other, as Christophe Boesch of the Swiss Center for Scientific Research notes. (Dr. Boesch makes this observation despite the fact that he and his wife, Hedwige Boesch, saw two rare instances of forest-dwelling chimpanzee mothers demonstrating nut-cracking techniques to their offspring.) According to Savage-Rumbaugh, apes seem to anticipate the actions of other apes or people, but they do not plan ahead as humans do, and they seem not to have an awareness of death.

Kathleen Gibson of the University of Texas Health Science Center[2] has also worked with chimpanzees and has a pet New World capuchin monkey who, like his conspecifics, is clever at using tools. She speculates that her pet could easily break a rock into flakes, but thinks that the monkey would never be able to put them back together again. Gibson believes that the act of putting things together sets people apart from nonhuman primates. Although it may not sound like much at first, a general ability to construct may, indeed, have far-reaching implications when it comes to putting together sentences or even generating ideas. Indeed, Gibson seems to have hit upon something very important here.

Chimpologists have a privileged perspective from which to compare the cognitive abilities of humans and apes. They are able to tell us certain ways in which humans are unique. Humans can attend to multiple tasks, cooperate, plan ahead, construct, and easily encode and transmit inventions to others. However, this list almost seems too narrow because as Savage-Rumbaugh observes, there is an enormous difference between chimpanzees and humans. Humans are just plain smarter. Both chimpanzees and young children use gestures combined with two-word utterances (pressing keys on the one hand, vocalizations on the other) to ask for cookies, tickles, games, favorite people, and so on. However, the chimpanzee never grows out of this stage. A human child always does. By five years of age, the child is capable of asking profound questions, but the chimpanzee is not. And, of course, spontaneous questions like "Mommy, where did I come from?" spring directly from the child's brain. That is the major difference between a chimpanzee and a human.

There is another general area of human accomplishment that chimpologists rarely mention, probably because it is so obvious. No chimpanzee ever wrote a book, composed a symphony, painted a realistic portrait, performed a *Singing in the Rain*–quality tap dance, calculated the day of the week upon which a certain date will fall next year, developed a math proof, took apart and reassembled a watch, programmed a computer, designed a bridge, or theorized about the origin of the universe. These arts and sciences also spring from special features of the human brain.

So what is it that the human brain has that the chimpanzee brain does not? Dissection of brains from each species has not provided an answer to this question. On a superficial level, brains of humans and brains of chimpanzees appear to have all the same parts. True, human brains are larger and more convoluted than chimpanzee brains. However, the other differences that exist

culus are noteworthy. For example, the sensory and motor maps of the left hemisphere represent the right side of the body, and vice versa (notice that both hands and both feet of the homunculus are from the right side of the body). Further, the sensory and motor maps for the opposite side of the body are *mirrored* around the central sulcus. Thus, sensory information for the *right* hand is received in the hand area behind the central sulcus of the *left* cerebral hemisphere, and the motor impulses to wiggle the fingers of the *right* hand come from the hand area in front of the central sulcus of the *left* hemisphere. Although there are exceptions, such crossed (or contralateral) representation is the general rule for the cerebral cortex.

The homunculus appears somewhat comical because of the distorted size of certain body parts, not to mention that it is upside down. However, for mammals in general, the size of the cortical area for a particular body part is a reflection of its functional importance in the day-to-day life of that animal. (Harry Jerison calls this the *principle of proper mass*.) The homunculus reflects the importance of hands and face for humans. Notice also that sensory and motor representations for the right foot curve over the top of the brain and extend down the (buried) inside surface of the hemisphere. Certain other interesting features are not shown in my homunculus. For example, sensory representation for genitals is located deep on the inside surface of the brain, near the sensory area for the foot. Similarly, sensory and motor representations for vocal structures such as the larynx and jaw are located right below the face representation (and just above the Sylvian fissure).

As shown in the first illustration, the Sylvian fissure separates the frontal and parietal lobes from the temporal lobe of the brain. Most of the primary auditory cortex (A) is located on the superior part of the temporal lobe and is buried within the floor of the Sylvian fissure. The primary auditory cortex is organized according to pitch of sounds and (contrary to the contralateral rule) receives substantial input from the ear of the same side, as well as a somewhat greater contribution from the opposite ear.

The primary visual area (V) is not always limited by the lunate sulcus in humans, as it is in other higher primates. The primary visual cortex is represented by just a small portion of the outside surface of the occipital lobe in humans, whereas larger areas are buried on the inside surfaces of the back of the brain. The right half of the visual field is represented in the primary visual cortex of the left hemisphere, and vice versa.

Each of the primary sensory areas has a special relationship with a nearby association area. For example, the primary somatosensory cortex (S) sends fibers to an area of the parietal lobe right behind it. Data from the general senses are integrated, related to past experiences, and interpreted in this association area. By way of illustration, it is this region that allows a person to interpret an unseen object held in the opposite hand as, say, a key. If the association cortex were damaged (but with the primary somatosensory cortex left intact), the individual would know that his hand held an object that was small, cold, and heavy. However, he would not be able to put the information together and arrive at the conclusion that the object was a key.

Similarly, the primary visual cortex (V) sends fibers to the association cortex right in front of it. In a manner like that just described for somatosensory association cortex, visual association cortex relates present to past visual experiences and permits recognition of what is seen and appreciation of its significance. Damage to this area results in an inability to recognize objects in the opposite visual field. The auditory association cortex (which is located right next to A) also permits the listener to recognize and interpret language and nonlanguage sounds.

The primary motor cortex has its helper too, called the premotor cortex. The premotor cortex is located directly in front of the primary motor cortex (and the homunculus). Stimulation of the premotor cortex causes muscle movements on the opposite side of the body, although stronger stimulation is required than for the primary motor cortex. The premotor cortex seems to be involved with accessing the memory of complex movements that have been learned (such as brushing the teeth), since these movements may be impaired by a lesion in that area, while other voluntary motor functions are spared.

There you have it: the basic cortical floorplan of higher primates including rhesus monkeys, chimpanzees, and humans. And it was probably the blueprint for the cortex of their common ancestor as well. But from whence the paintings, the symphonies, the great books? Those came with nature's elaborations of three overlapping cortical features whose seeds were sown long before the world saw its first hominid: the frontal lobes, association cortex, and brain lateralization.

Inner Models of Reality
Domain of the Frontal Lobes

The area in front of the premotor cortex (i.e., the foremost end of the frontal lobe) is known as the prefrontal association cortex. Unlike primary motor and premotor cortices, bodily movements are not usually elicited when the prefrontal cortex is stimulated. Thus, the prefrontal cortex is said to be silent. Silent it may be, but a lot is going on there nevertheless. For it is the prefrontal cortex that is responsible for self-regulated, goal-directed behaviors that are formative of personality. In some sense, then, it is the prefrontal cortex that makes us human.

Not too many years ago, it was considered appropriate to treat severe depression (often in housewives) by removing part of the prefrontal cortex or by severing the tracts that connect it with other, deeper parts of the brain. Although such prefrontal lobotomies did cure patients of depression, they also resulted in a host of less-desirable changes. To greater or lesser degrees (depending on the amount of brain damage sustained), frontal lobe patients were subject to thought disorders, inappropriate or generally flattened moods, lack of initiative, poverty of speech, and inability to grasp the significance of events going on around them. Prefrontal lobotomies were also used to treat intractable pain, such as that associated with inoperable cancer. In these cases, although patients could still experience pain after their surgeries, they no longer minded it! Prefrontal lobotomies thus resulted in nothing less than complete personality changes.

Frontal lobes expanded greatly during primate evolution. In particular, compared with more posterior regions of the brain, the prefrontal cortex is much more convoluted in humans than in apes.[5] Even in monkeys, the prefrontal cortex is highly differentiated and has multiple subdivisions and connections. Because the prefrontal cortex of macaques is relatively well understood, the neuroanatomy of this species provides insights that may shed light on the basic floorplan and evolutionary significance of the human frontal lobe.

Patricia Goldman-Rakic, of Yale University School of Medicine, has incorporated a good deal of experimental evidence on macaques into an elegant model that explains much about the basic organization of the primate prefrontal cortex.[6] According to Goldman-Rakic, the elemental capacity of the prefrontal cortex is to access information and keep it on-line (i.e., in mind) until the task at hand is completed. It can also stimulate or inhibit motor responses based on the on-line representation. Thus, the prefrontal cortex affects attention, accessing memories, and governing behavior via motor control.

Further, because of their connections to other lobes as well as deeper brain structures, specific areas of the prefrontal cortex seem to specialize in the types of information they process. One part of the prefrontal cortex of macaques holds on-line the positions of objects in space, while another attends to nonspatial visual attributes of objects, such as color. Although not as well understood, still another area of the monkey prefrontal cortex may be associated with social/emotional and motivational states. In sum, Goldman-Rakic hypothesizes that "the subdivisions of the primate prefrontal cortex function as central executive centers for guiding voluntary behavior by representational memory."[7] Put another way, the prefrontal cortex integrates events that are separated in time and space and uses stored representational knowledge to guide appropriate responses. Without it, neither monkey nor man could keep enough information in mind to plan even a little bit ahead.

Of course, humans are the supreme planners. A chimpanzee can hold on-line the location of previously stored food and go for it when permitted to do so. However, Savage-Rumbaugh tells us that unlike humans, chimpanzees have difficulty attending to more than one task at a time, do not plan much ahead, and seem to have no concept of death (perhaps the ultimate in planning ahead). Because it has expanded so much during hominid evolution, the frontal lobe is the one part of the brain in which chimpanzee and human sulcal patterns are easily distinguishable. And along with expanded size of the human frontal lobe came an elaboration of the capacities that Goldman-Rakic has enumerated for the prefrontal cortex of nonhuman primates.

The human frontal lobe not only brings information on-line, presumably it can bring lots of information on-line simultaneously. Thus, the prefrontal cortex of humans may access relatively more memory to guide voluntary motor responses than is the case for nonhuman primates. An increased capacity to bring memory on-line would account, in part, for the fact that learned motor behaviors of humans can entail longer sequences of activity that are more finely controlled than those of apes. (Recall that the performance of learned motor skills is associated with the premotor cortex, which presumably is influenced by the prefrontal cortex.) As a result, people learn intricate, sequential motor activities that are uniquely and gloriously human, such as (my favorite) tap dancing.

Tap dancing depends, first and foremost, on a kind of motor memory, and second, on the ability to smoothly execute a sequence of learned movements (taps) that are remembered. Rhythm, or timing, is everything—botch the spacing between taps, and you ruin the dance. In order to perform, a tap dancer must be able to actualize the memory of how to correctly time taps. This requires anticipation of what is ahead. The tap dancer's holding of representations of long motor sequences on-line long enough to execute them correctly bridges time noticeably. The tap dance has a past, present, and future. And so, alas, does the tap dancer. Whereas chimpanzees can only plan a bit ahead (get that food bait), thanks to its evolved frontal lobes, the species that tap dances has a conscious concept of time.

Another unique human characteristic that may be attributed

to elaborate frontal lobes is an active imagination. Because of their ability to time bind, people can hold real or fictitious ideas on-line and spin all kinds of scenarios. We've all relived unpleasant past events and imagined "if only I'd done such and such." In the face of frustrating past (or present) events, one may entertain other outcomes and obtain satisfaction after all, if only in the mind's eye. Perhaps more important, an active fantasy life allows humans to anticipate variations of future events and imagine (practice) alternate responses. The human imagination is so powerful that it cannot sit still. If it's not being used for something practical or being occupied (e.g., by television), it will entertain itself with gratuitous fantasies. Apparently, the frontal lobe provides its own entertainment center. And, as dreams show, its doors are unlocked twenty-four hours a day.

Perhaps the most mysterious function of the frontal lobe has to do with personality factors, such as individual styles of social awareness and behaviors toward others. Chimpanzees do not show the same degree of frontal-lobe mediated self-regulation of responses to social/emotional events as mature humans do. Human frontal lobes have complex connections with other deeper parts of the brain (known as limbic structures) that are concerned with emotional processes. Thus, codes of conduct that have been deeply ingrained in childhood may be accessed and represented in the prefrontal cortex and, ultimately, brought to bear on adult social interactions. Mature people attempt to govern their social interactions and to take other individuals into account (i.e., to guard against childish behavior).

Higher Thought Processes: The Association Areas

A synthesis of neurological events, or gluing together of information that occurs in the frontal lobes, is a form of thinking. And the prefrontal association cortex is not the only part of the brain that transforms multiple inputs into higher-order thoughts. This kind of synthetic thinking also occurs in other association areas of the temporal, parietal, and occipital lobes. One way to get a handle on the general functions of these posterior association areas is to examine the intriguing syndromes that occur in people when these areas are damaged.[8] For example, we've already noted that damage to the association regions contiguous with the primary receptive areas interferes with the integration and interpretation of sensory information. Thus, if a lesion occurs in the area that is directly in front of the primary visual cortex, a person will walk around an obstacle such as a ladder (indicating that he sees it), yet be unable to name it, say what it is used for, or point out that he has just avoided bad luck. In short, the visual input is there, but the ability to interpret it is not.

Sensations of touch, hearing, and vision are integrated in the parietal association cortex. Because of connections between the parietal association cortex and other areas such as the frontal lobes, these complex associations are interpreted in light of past experience and present judgment. Damage to parietal association areas can therefore lead to bizarre dysfunctions; the best known entails a failure to recognize body scheme. A person (or nonhuman primate) with this syndrome does not recognize a part of his body as belonging to himself. For example, if the damaged area of the parietal lobe is the association cortex for the hand (of the opposite side of the body), the individual does not recognize the hand as his own. He will not talk about the hand, wash it, or put a glove on it. He does, however, know that the hand is a hand and may in fact be quite frightened of it because, to him, it is someone else's hand. This same neglect syndrome occurs for other parts of the body such as the face, depending on which parts of the superior parietal lobe are damaged.

The sense of our own whole bodies is so intrinsic to our day-to-day living that we do not ordinarily think of this experience as being dependent upon synthetic neurological processes. Yet it is. And just as we all have an awareness of our body scheme, we also have an awareness of visuospatial relationships in the external world. Along with expanded association areas, visuospatial skills, or the related ability to map one's environment, are especially well developed in humans. The extent of these skills varies with sex (males outperform females on some tests) and from individual to individual. Certain visuospatial abilities are also better developed on the right side of the brain.

Olfactory, auditory, and visual associations dominate the front part of the temporal lobe. These associations are influenced by other parts of the brain, including the frontal lobe, a nearby limbic area on the underside of the temporal lobe that is important for memory (the hippocampus), and other limbic structures that are concerned with emotions. Consequently, the association cortex of the front part of the temporal lobe is susceptible to its own interesting syndrome. Damage to this area results in vivid auditory, visual, or olfactory hallucinations. For example, a temporal lobe patient may experience a strong sense of déjà vu, while hearing distorted music that is not there or seeing hallucinations of funny little (or large) people. Depending on the size of the area involved, the person may also smell nonexistent disagreeable odors and experience intense, irrational fear. A dreamy sense of unreality often accompanies these hallucinations, and the patient frequently realizes that the sensations are not real.

Remove the temporal lobes in human and nonhuman primates, and a suite of similar symptoms occur in what is known as the Kluver-Bucy syndrome. These symptoms include psychic blindness, a tendency to examine everything with the mouth, voracious appetite, increased sexual activity, marked absence of emotional responses, and general docility. Although it is unlikely that a temporal-lobe-damaged monkey ever hallucinated music, the Kluver-Bucy syndrome suggests that, once again, temporal-lobe association areas of humans are elaborations woven from a basic primate floorplan.

Language Areas: Manifestation of a Lateralized Brain

Over a century ago, Paul Broca discovered an amazing fact from postmortem autopsies of patients with speech disorders. Their brains almost invariably had damage in a specific area of the left hemisphere. Today, we know that language has both sensory and motor components. It is therefore represented by two distinct areas in the brain, one posterior and one anterior. The sensory area for *comprehension* of spoken words (known as Wernicke's area) is next to the primary auditory area in the temporal lobe. The motor area for *speech* (Broca's area) is located in the frontal lobe near the primary motor areas that stimulate the organs of speech (e.g., larynx, tongue, mouth). As anticipated by Broca's initial discovery, both language areas are located in the left hemisphere. Although they are on the same side of the brain, damage to these areas results in different types of aphasias.

Patients with Broca's aphasia are fine in the comprehension department. However, they have great difficulty speaking or writing what they wish to say. Their speech is terribly slow and, when it finally comes, is characterized by poor articulation. Although patients may be able to produce single meaningful words, small words and endings are usually omitted. As a result, their sentences (such as they are) are grammatically incorrect. Left-hemisphere damage may extend to the primary motor cortex, which accounts for the fact that Broca's aphasiacs also frequently experience paralysis of the right side of the body.

Wernicke's aphasia is quite a different story. Although a patient's basic hearing abilities may be unimpaired, comprehension of speech is severely disrupted by damage to Wernicke's area. (If the damage is extended posteriorly, reading ability will also be lost.) Because Broca's area is undamaged, the rhythm and grammatical scaffolding of speech appear normal. Verbal output seems effortless in Wernicke's patients, yet its content is full of numerous errors, including lots of little words and circumlocutions. In short, speech has little meaning in the Wernicke's aphasiac. It is "word salad."

The above summaries of Broca's and Wernicke's aphasias are, of course, oversimplifications. Beneath the surface of the cortex, the two areas of the brain connect with each other and with other cortical areas. There are not only two types of aphasia but also many different manifestations (each with unique combinations of symptoms). Perhaps more important, the left-hemisphere areas

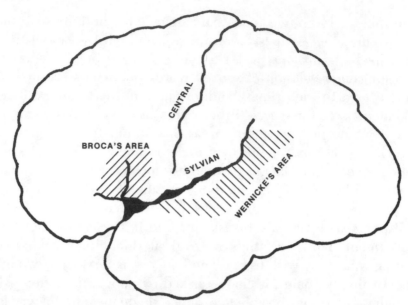

The left hemisphere of a human brain showing Broca's speech area (in front) and Wernicke's area (in rear).

for comprehension and production of language extend beyond those that have been classically defined. In some sense, both Broca's area and Wernicke's area should be larger than shown in my illustration. Although Wernicke didn't know it, his area should extend back up and around the end of the Sylvian fissure, because it is here that reading and a full understanding of the symbolism of language are facilitated.[9] Likewise, Broca's area should be extended forward to include part of the area that is directly in front of it.[10]

Because language so dramatically separates humans from nonhuman primates, the evolutionary importance of Broca's and Wernicke's areas has been greatly emphasized. Do nonhuman primates have these areas? The answer is yes and no. Yes, there are frontal lobe and temporal/parietal regions in the brains of monkeys and apes that appear to be in (somewhat) similar positions and to have similar arrangements of cells as Broca's and Wernicke's areas do in human brains. There is also some evidence that the left hemisphere differentially processes socially meaningful vocalizations in nonhuman higher primates. It therefore appears that, once again, human language areas are an elaboration on the basic primate pattern. However, the sulcal pattern associated with Broca's area in humans does not appear in the hominid fossil record until two million years ago. And of course, monkeys and apes don't talk or read books.

Body Language

Because of its predilection for language, the left hemisphere is known as the major hemisphere. During development, the left hemisphere matures more slowly than the right hemisphere. And some workers believe that the left hemisphere was a kind of late bloomer during primate evolution as well (i.e., that it changed more than the right hemisphere during hominid evolution). All of this credit has gone to the left hemisphere because of one package of skills—those related to language.

I believe that the above interpretation is too narrow. We have toured the different lobes of the brain and have seen numerous ways in which humans differ cognitively from their chimpanzee (and monkey) cousins. Yes, the left hemisphere of the human brain is particularly good at analytical, time-sequencing processes that are important for language. As we have seen, it can count (keep time) and smoothly execute strings of ordered motor events. And the left hemisphere can bring past experience online and use it to influence not only what is said, but also what is done. Contrary to popular wisdom, then, human beings apply the analytical, sequencing skills of the left hemisphere to the task of communicating with their *whole bodies*, rather than with just their vocal anatomies. Language is important, but it is not everything.

Take, for instance, the gesticulation that accompanies speech. When people talk, so do their bodies: Heads bob, arms flail, eyebrows are raised, and hands go everywhere. Further, these bodily movements are rhythmically coordinated with speech. As Adam Kendon, a leading expert on gesture, puts it: "Speech and movement appear together, as manifestations of the same process of utterance. That is, in the translation of 'ideas' into observable behavior . . . the output that results is manifested in both speech and movement."[11] Kendon observes that the starting point that leads to generation of a multifaceted utterance is its semantic organization. It is the underlying meaning that drives communication.

As we speak, most of us are barely aware of our gesticulations. It is therefore surprising to learn that the gesticulations that accompany speech are not only planned, but are planned prior to the spoken phrase with which they concur. Apparently, the analytical frontal lobe sequencing machinery plans ahead, coordinates, and executes all kinds of motor activities in its mission to express meaning. By way of example, Kendon offers the following beautiful description from a videotape recording of a woman telling a fairy tale:

> The speaker is recounting how the hunter rescued Little Red Riding Hood's grandmother from the Big Bad Wolf, who had just eaten her. The speaker says: "And he took his hatchet and with a mighty sweep, sliced the wolf's stomach open." . . . As the speaker says "sliced" she brings both her hands down from an upraised position, sweeping them to her left as she does so, in what is clearly an enactment of the hunter's action. However, to do this, the speaker had to have her hands positioned in advance of the word "sliced." She organizes her hands into an upraised position as she says "and he took his hatchet," actually beginning this process before she begins to speak at all, and she holds her hands upraised while she says "and with a mighty sweep."
>
> . . . In the example given, for instance, it will be clear that the enactment of the hunter's action and the account given in speech must have been organized simultaneously. An image of the hunter's action must have been available before the speaker embarked on her speech. Note, further, that the speaker, having raised her arms in preparation for the slicing movement, does not perform it at once, but waits until she has

reached the word "sliced." The placement of the stroke of the gesture phrase (in this case the "slicing" enactment, that is) in relation to the verbal representation of the action described is thus an organized placement. The conjoint deployment of the two modes of representation seen here, in which the stroke of the gesture phrase is timed to fit with the structure of the spoken passage, must itself be seen as part of the utterance plan.

In the example just discussed, the speaker adjusted the performance of her gesture to fit with the structure of the concurrent speech phrase. In other instances we may observe the reverse of this: the speaker adjusts the production of speech to the performance of gesture. This further strengthens the point that gesture and speech are produced conjointly, as integral parts of a single utterance plan.[12]

This example illustrates that gesticulation and speech work together to communicate meaning in a subtle but complex manner. However, as Kendon points out, the mode of encoding content is different in the two forms of expression. In speech, highly conventionalized forms from an established vocabulary are organized sequentially and according to grammatical rules. On the other hand, although conventionalized forms may be used in gesticulation, the utterer has considerable leeway to create new gestures and to form constructions that are relatively free of grammatical constraints. Susan Goldin-Meadow of the University of Chicago has shown that, interestingly, children who are born deaf organize gestures into a fully linguistic system.[13] Thus, gesticulation retains its free spirit only if the utterer has access to both speech and gestural modes of expression.

What area of the brain facilitates gesticulation? We know that people who are right-handed (and left-hemisphere dominant for language) gesticulate more with that hand than with the left. It is also known that stimulation of the primary cortical (motor) hand representation causes the hand on the opposite side of the body to move, just as stimulation of primary facial and vocal areas causes movement of these structures. During speech, Broca's area somehow facilitates proper functioning of the primary motor cortex that controls the vocal anatomy. But what cortical areas influence primary hand representations? Does the frontal-lobe association cortex that is next to the primary hand region (above Broca's area) act as a kind of Broca's area, but for the hand? Perhaps it does.

Whatever the details of their neurological underpinnings, speech and gesticulation flow effortlessly together in order to achieve the mutual goal of expressing ideas that are brought online (represented) in the frontal lobes. Indeed, the two modes of communication can be difficult to separate, as illustrated by a well known interesting fact about simultaneous translators. Apparently, simultaneous translation of one language into another is a thoroughly exhausting enterprise. It is said that translators frequently occupy their hands with some rote activity such as knitting. Presumably, this minimizes the distraction that would ensue from attempting to gesticulate in concurrence with two slightly differently paced languages!

Chimpanzees Can't Tap Dance

As far as I am concerned, cortical areas for feet also have access to a kind of Broca's area (if not *the* Broca's area). I say this for the simple reason that I took tap lessons for five years and found this activity not only to be linguistic, but also one in which no chimpanzee could ever skillfully engage. Tap dancing, like speech, entails production of finely coordinated motor sequences that are based on an accepted vocabulary of smaller units. It is hierarchically organized and is generated according to grammatical rules. The left hemisphere prevails, since most tappers are better on their right sides. As with any foreign language, little kids learn tap easily, while adults have to struggle.

My tap class was taught by Cynthea Riffle, a professional dancer who taught ballet, tap, and jazz dance for a number of years in San Juan, Puerto Rico. She began taking tap lessons at age seven and by ten was also studying ballet, jazz, voice, and piano.

For five years, Cynthea taught tap classes to six middle-aged adults who met once a week in her studio. (As an ecologist in the group put it, "You have to do something to keep in touch with your culture.") We were lucky to have a teacher who was incredibly fluent in tap. It was like taking lessons from Ginger Rogers.[14]

Cynthea's tap dancing is primarily an activity of her left hemisphere. Her dancing may be thought of as a kind of speech of the feet. Her right hemisphere is also involved, of course, since it controls the left side of her body. But it is the left hemisphere that is keeping time and running the show. It does so by sending instructions to Cynthea's right hemisphere. These precisely timed instructions are transmitted over nerve fibers that cross to the right hemisphere through a large C-shaped structure known as the corpus callosum. The corpus callosum is simply a big bundle of fibers that connects the two halves of the brain.

Despite the above observations about tap dancing, traffic along the corpus callosum is not one-way. Furthermore, the much beleaguered right hemisphere is often in the driver's seat. In fact, this has probably been the case since the days of the first primates. Contrary to popular wisdom, I believe that it was the right, rather than the left, hemisphere that drove the evolution of brain lateralization. (This will be discussed later.)

Although they are very smart, even the most educated chimpanzees are not able to tap dance. Signing chimpanzees instead use their hard-won language skills almost exclusively to seek food or other immediate gratification. We pride ourselves that, by comparison, human intellectual and artistic achievements are so great that they must be the result of qualitative improvements in the human nervous system. According to this line of thought, it is not just that humans have more brains than chimpanzees, but also that humans have better brains. As we have seen, comparative neuroanatomists speculate that the neurological basis for the difference in consciousness between the chimpanzee and the human child is based on evolutionary improvements in three features: the frontal lobes, association cortices, and brain lateralization.

But at what point during hominid evolution did these changes begin?

We know that australopithecine endocasts were about the size of chimpanzee brains and that, superficially, the pattern of their convolutions appeared apelike. However, because of allometric scaling, the latter is exactly what one would expect in light of the former. But australopithecines were not apes. Rather, they were ape-men who occupied their own unique niches. It is therefore safe to surmise from the fossil record and from comparative neuroanatomical studies that australopithecines would have had at least the cognitive ability of chimpanzees—and perhaps more.

Of course, the most striking feature about australopithecines was that they walked upright. I believe that selection for bipedalism in early gracile australopithecines kicked off the train of events that would eventually lead to even more advanced brains. Bipedalism is the key to understanding human brain evolution.

In his essay, Malthus pointed out that if human populations are unrestrained by natural causes, they will double in size every twenty-five years. He also claimed that food production increased linearly and that it therefore could not keep up with the geometric increase in population size. Malthus concluded that the struggle for existence kept animal populations in check, but that artificial restraints would have to be applied to humans. It was specifically the notion of natural checks on population size that excited the imaginations of Darwin and Wallace.[2]

Darwin and Wallace independently had the same "aha" experience after reading Malthus's essay. They realized that those individuals with characteristics that were the most favorable for survival (individuals who were the best adapted) would prevail over others in the struggle for existence. It was that simple. In 1859, Darwin went on to elaborate this theory of evolution in his book *On the Origin of Species by Means of Natural Selection, or the Preservation of Favoured Races in the Struggle for Life*.

Darwin's theory can be reiterated in a sequence of logical steps. First, because of Malthus, Darwin assumed that *all* species produced more offspring than could be fed; therefore only some individuals of each species would survive. Second, the survivors would naturally turn out to be those who were better adapted to their particular environments—the stronger, the quicker, and the like. A very important third assumption was that favorable traits of those who survived could be inherited by the next generation. (Darwin knew this was true, although he was not familiar with Gregor Mendel's work on genes.) Darwin concluded that entirely new species resulted from the above processes acting over long periods of geological time. Today, traditional and molecular evolutionists may quibble about the pace, rates, and methods for studying evolution, but Darwin's grand theory still stands.

Our Arboreal Heritage

In an exciting recent development, the brunt of the molecular evidence now suggests that humans share a more recent common ancestor (CA) with chimpanzees than with any other primate, including gorillas. (In fact, the genetic similarity between chimpanzees and humans is so close that some workers have suggested that a cross between a human and a chimpanzee might theocratically be possible!) Furthermore, molecular anthropologists have determined that the CA lived about five million years ago, an estimate which traditional anthropologists find they can live with.[3]

Although all known fossil hominids were bipedal, we know that at some point they, like our cousins, the chimpanzees, had ancestors who were arboreal. Thus, the CA bequeathed certain general arboreal primate traits to early chimpanzees and our early hominid relatives. Simply put, although hominids lived on the ground and walked on two legs, many of the features that they inherited were developed over millions of years of primate evolution *in trees*. This is a basic theme in primatology and is called the "Arboreal Theory."[4] It also applies to humans.

Look in the mirror and you will see a primate who retains many adaptations for life in the trees. Those eyes. They face forward, instead of sideways like a dog's. All the better to see with in three dimensions (a result of the two eyes' visual fields overlapping). And seeing in three dimensions is very helpful when it comes to leaping around in a complicated environment that is up high. What shoulders. They're sturdy and allow a good deal of mobility in the upper arms. A necessity for suspending one's weight by the arms or swinging through trees.

Look at your hands. They have really good grasping ability and fingernails instead of claws. Hands like these are great for hanging onto branches without clawing oneself in the palms. The hands and eyes together make for good hand-eye coordination in primates. This is useful for picking, inspecting, and eating plant food. Or for catching insects. No snout. Many of its grasping functions (including picking food) were taken over by hands in an arboreal environment. Further, the keen sense of smell that is associated with a snout is not as important as good vision for a tree-living primate.

Besides these physical features, we also inherited certain related behaviors from our distant tree-living ancestors. For example, we sleep in beds that derive from tree nests. During the night, people sometimes awaken briefly with a quick jerk. Fear of falling from the nest? How do you regard snakes or spiders? These creatures evoke terror in many humans, and I suspect we owe this oddity to our arboreal legacy, as well. Chimpanzees apparently select their lodge trees and construct their night nests with an eye toward avoiding just such dangers. (I avoid these and other frights by pulling the covers up over my body before going to sleep.)

Some of our daytime activities are also rooted in the trees. Children at playgrounds love to do arboreal acrobatics (playing on the bars). Adults also have the ability to swing through the trees. However, except for joining sports programs or the circus, there is little opportunity to develop this proclivity in our culture. In one respect, hand-eye coordination is important to us in much the same way that it is to an arboreal primate—we visually inspect our food before bringing it to our mouth. If it looks questionable, we either do not put it into our mouth or do so knowing that we may regret it later. Primates, including ourselves, would be truly miserable eating blindfolded.

So these traits are part of the general primate baggage that was handed down to the CA of chimpanzees and humans some five million years ago. We should also include good mothering, a tendency for child's play and, of course, a lively curiosity. The latter is very important and goes with another special feature that developed during primate evolution—an unusually large brain.

Getting the Feet on the Ground

But what set the CA apart from other primates? Unfortunately, there are no fossil hominids from five million years ago. One can, therefore, only guess on the basis of later fossil hominids and living apes. Adrienne Zihlman, professor of anthropology at the University of California, Santa Cruz, has done comparative studies of ape anatomy and fossil hominid bones which have led her to one of the best assessments going for the CA. Unfortunately, and predictably, she has not always been given due credit for her contribution. Zihlman candidly discusses the frustrations of doing paleoanthropological research, noting that any successful new hypothesis passes through three predictable stages on the road to respectability:

> First, it is criticized for being untrue.
>
> Secondly, after supporting evidence accumulates, it is stated that it may be true, but it is not particularly relevant.
>
> Thirdly, after it has clearly influenced the field, it is admitted to be true and relevant, but the same critics assert that the idea was not original.[5]

As Zihlman details, this progression is exactly what happened to her pygmy-chimpanzee hypothesis.

According to the Zihlman model, the CA resembled pygmy chimpanzees (bonobos) more than any other living primates, including the common chimpanzees one usually sees in zoos. Zihlman points out that bonobos are relatively small, with long arms and especially long legs. Of all the apes, pygmy chimpanzees come closest to resembling the earliest fossil hominids (such as Lucy) in terms of general body build. They also seem to be the most like humans in their social and sexual behavior.

Bonobos have a peculiar way of getting about on the ground, a form of locomotion that they share with the common chimpanzee and gorilla. They frequently walk on all fours. But the hands are doubled over (palms down) so that the forward weight is placed on the knuckles rather than the palms when they walk. This form of locomotion, known as knuckle-walking, is just plain weird among primates and is thought to have resulted when the tree-living ancestors of chimpanzees and gorillas (with long hands for hanging onto branches) took to the ground. Thus, the formerly clinging hand became a weight-bearing structure and tucked its fingers out of the way in the process. Bonobos don't always knuckle-walk. They sometimes stand up and walk bipedally, although with more of a bent knee and bent hip than humans have

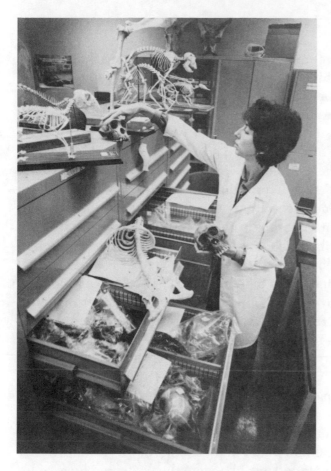

Adrienne Zihlman. Her comparative studies of ape anatomy and fossil hominid bones provide important evidence for understanding certain aspects of the earliest hominids. (Courtesy University of California, Santa Cruz)

when they walk. Bonobos are even known to walk bipedally along tree branches, especially if they are carrying food.

Because knuckle-walking is present in both gorillas and chimpanzees, some paleoanthropologists believe that the common ancestor of hominids and chimpanzees must also have been a knuckle-walker. Others reject this idea because fossil hominids and living humans do not show any vestiges of knuckle-walking in their hand bones. Perhaps the arboreal ancestors of the CA resembled pygmy chimpanzees in having a tendency toward bipedalism, both in the trees and on the ground. As the CA shifted toward spending a significant portion of time on the ground, knuckle-walking may have developed only in its ape descendants who took the quadrupedal route. Unlike the situation for chimpanzees, however, the tendency toward bipedalism eventually won out over that for quadrupedalism in the hominid descendants of the CA. Thus, full-fledged knuckle-walking may not have developed in the CA, but only in some of its descendants. This would explain the absence of signs of knuckle-walking in the hands of early fossil hominids and ourselves.

But, there is an objection to this reasoning. If knuckle-walking did not occur in the common ancestor of chimpanzees and hominids, then chimpanzees acquired this habit *after* their separation from hominids some five million years ago. Since gorillas seem to have split off from CA stock several million years earlier, they would have come by this unusual mode of locomotion independently. Some paleoanthropologists think that this would be too much of a coincidence. So take your pick: Was the common ancestor of chimpanzees and hominids a knuckle-walker or not? I don't know for sure, but, if not, the ancestors of hominids may never have gotten to a knuckle-walking stage because they literally walked away from it![6]

Yet, whatever form of locomotion characterized the common ancestor of chimpanzees and hominids, one thing is for sure. Since all known fossil hominids were bipeds, walking on two legs probably played an important role in the origin of the hominid family some five million years ago. Furthermore, I believe that the question of why bipedalism became the preferred form of locomotion in early hominids remains one of the biggest unsolved mysteries in hominid paleontology.

Footprints in Time

The hominid fossil record is precious. Hominids become fossilized only under special circumstances—when minerals such as calcite or silica are deposited within the bones or teeth of dead individuals. Through time, cavities that were previously empty or filled with soft tissue absorb more minerals from the burial environment. The fossil bone or tooth becomes harder and heavier. Usually, the fossil just sits there quietly like a rock, never to be discovered. Occasionally, however, fossilized teeth or fragments of bone are collected or unearthed by archaeologists or paleontologists. But this is a rare event. That is why fossil hominids are priceless and are kept locked away in bank vaults.

The fossil record of our early hominid ancestors picks up about 3.5 million years ago, with a remarkable discovery from Laetoli, Tanzania, announced by Mary Leakey in 1978.[7] Thousands of fossilized footprints of animals had been discovered. Pigs, elephants, giraffes, hyenas, antelopes, horses, and rhinoceroses were among the many species that left tracks at Laetoli. So were hominids who, by this time, had experienced a million and a half years of evolution since splitting from the ancestors of chimpanzees.

Three hominids had walked slowly north across the grassy savanna. The ground was covered with a layer of ash from a nearby active volcano, and it was damp at the time of their walk (perhaps from rain). Think of it as walking on the beach, next to the water, as the tide goes out. Footprints are left in the wet sand, and these become crusted or set as the sand dries. The same thing happened at Laetoli. But with one difference. The tide never returned to erase the Laetoli footprints. Instead, the tracks were covered and preserved by more ashes from the volcano. Over time, they became fossilized.

Three and a half million years later, these hominid footprints were studied by Russell Tuttle, of the University of Chicago.[8] He estimated that the shortest hominid in the group was about four feet tall. Another who was about four feet, ten inches walked to the right of the first hominid. A third individual overprinted and partially obscured the tracks of the second; he was apparently taller still. Were the hominids walking together or separately? Could the second and third individuals have been following the first "with lust, murder, or other mayhem in mind," as Tuttle so vividly wondered? According to Tuttle, the answers to these questions, as well as certain other specifics about the Laetoli hominids, remain unknown. Nevertheless, the Laetoli footprints have much to tell.

Tuttle has convincingly argued that the Laetoli footprints are virtually indistinguishable from those made by small *Homo*

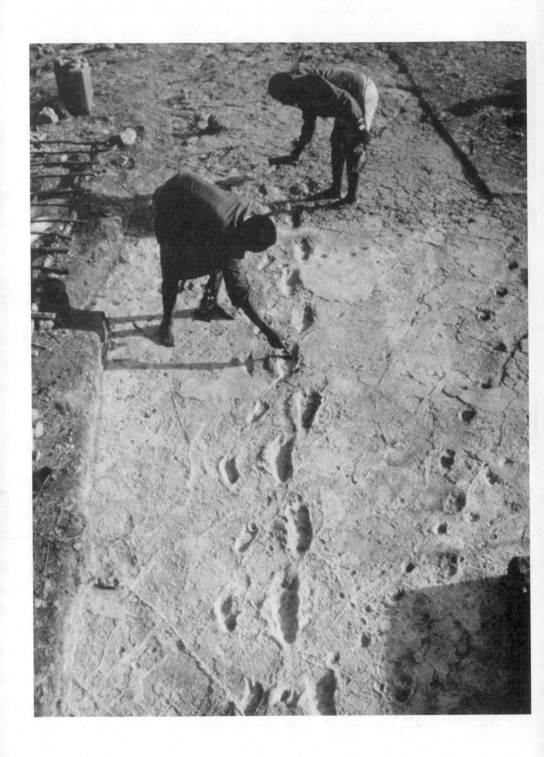

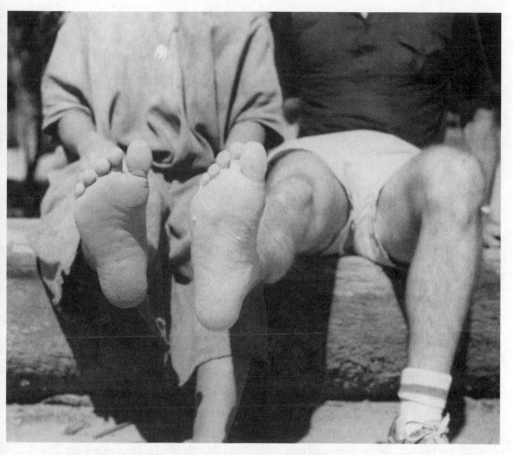

Right soles of a never-shod fourteen-year-old Machiguenga Indian male (left) and of habitually shod Russell Tuttle (right). Tuttle has convincingly argued that the Laetoli footprints are virtually indistinguishable from those made by small Homo sapiens who do not wear shoes. (Photograph courtesy Russell Tuttle)

(Opposite page) A trail of hominid footprints that were fossilized in volcanic ash was discovered at Laetoli, Tanzania. The trail shows that 3.5 million years ago some hominids were already bipedal. (Photograph by John Reader, copyright © 1992/Science Photo Library)

sapiens who are not used to wearing shoes. The big toes of the Laetoli hominids were aligned alongside the other toes, instead of sticking out from the foot like the big toes of apes. And Laetoli toes appear, like ours, to have been less curved than those of apes.[9] Laetoli feet had good arches—a must for efficiently supporting and shifting the weight of the body while walking on two legs. Most telling of all, the depths of certain parts of the footprints (e.g., the big toes and heels) show that the Laetoli hominids shifted their weight across their feet in *exactly* the same pattern that characterizes humans when they are walking. Although the Laetoli footprints are just whispered impressions left in the sands of time, the information they convey is extremely important. By 3.5 million years ago, at least *some* hominids were completely bipedal.

Bipedalism, more than anything else, separates early hominids from apes. Yet the primary cause for bipedalism remains the biggest unsolved mystery in hominid paleontology. However, it's not for lack of discussion in the literature. Speculation abounds. So, too, does controversy. Some workers argue that bipedalism occurred more or less in one fell swoop (a sort of "quick and dirty" school of thought). Others believe that full bipedalism was achieved more slowly during the course of hominid evolution. There is even a battle-of-the-sexes contingent among students of bipedalism. Was bipedalism selected for mainly in males or females? Each sex has its advocates.

The Laetoli footprints invalidated an important theory of bipedalism. I call this recently deceased theory the "2001" model, in honor of the wonderful opening sequence from the movie of the same name. The "2001" theory was a cyclical one, in which the evolution of bipedalism and of the brain occurred more or less simultaneously: Bipedalism freed the forelimbs, the freed hands made tools, tool production selected for intelligence, and greater intelligence caused bigger brains that produced still better tools.[10] This model captured the imaginations of anthropologists for many years, but was eventually doomed by the discovery that the earliest known hominids, although bipedal, had small, ape-size cranial capacities (and therefore small brains). As the fossil

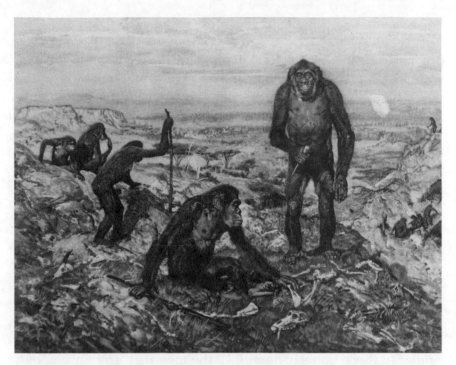

This 1970 drawing of australopithecines (species undetermined), demonstrates that the "2001" theory had captured the imagination of anthropologists. (Courtesy Department of Library Services, American Museum of Natural History)

record now reveals, the increase in brain size did not take off until a million and a half years after the first whispers of bipedalism at Laetoli.[11] The same is true for the production of stone tools. Thanks in large part to the footprints from Laetoli, bipedalism has been thoroughly disengaged from both brain size and tool production.

Then why did early hominids become bipedal? Most of the causes that have recently been proposed for bipedalism fall into two simple categories: food and sex. Of the two, the acquisition of food has received more attention. But what kind of food? Animal food or plant food? As has occurred among contemporary American consumers, paleoanthropology has had its own food fads. At the moment, meat is out and vegetables are in (on both fronts).

Not many years ago, the notion of man the hunter had an important role in theories about bipedalism. Early hominid men were out hunting while females and children remained at the home base. For physiological reasons having to do with breathing, bipedalism would have been adaptive for long-distance running after game (so-called persistence hunting), as well as for freeing the hands to make hunting weapons and to carry meat home. This theory tied in well with the "2001" model.[12] And the bottom line was that males made the tools and brought home the bacon. At least they did until (mostly) female anthropologists pointed out the obvious.

Woman the Gatherer

In modern hunting and gathering societies that live in habitats similar to those of early hominids, the men may go hunting, but, on a day-to-day basis, it is the women who end up providing most of the nourishment for the entire group. While *he* is out trying his luck at hunting, *she* (often accompanied by children) collects the more widely available plant food, insects, and small animals. She ensures that neither her children nor her hunter will go hungry tonight!

According to this woman-the-gatherer hypothesis, not only did early hominid women provide most of the food, but their freed forelimbs may have fashioned the first tools.[13] What did they use these tools for? To acquire food—by digging it up, knocking it down, or cracking something open. (With regard to the last, it is interesting that female chimpanzees appear to be more adept than male chimpanzees at cracking open nuts with rocks.[14]) Natural selection for bipedalism would have been especially strong for gathering mothers. Accordingly, early hominid women may have invented slings or other devices with which to carry small children and containers for food or water.

"Man" the hunter has suffered other affronts. Carnivores such as lions or hyenas are known to leave tooth marks on the bones of animals they eat. Similarly, early hominids sometimes left their own stamp, in the form of cut marks, on the bones of animals they butchered with stone tools. Relatively recent studies by paleontologist and science writer Pat Shipman have examined the layering of hominid cut marks and carnivore tooth marks on animal bones associated with early hominid sites.[15] And guess what? More often than not, our intrepid hunter got there after the kill. It may well have been man the scavenger instead of man the hunter. (And one of his earliest inventions may have been the fish story, as he explained how he caught the big one that got away!)

In 1981, Owen Lovejoy of Kent State University offered a kinder, gentler picture of the early male hominid. He did so by suggesting a unique man-the-gatherer theory to explain the origin of bipedalism.[16] According to Lovejoy, early hominids were near the brink of extinction. He therefore sought to identify some aspect of bipedalism that would have increased the number of living offspring of early hominids. Because food, water, and sleeping trees were widely scattered in the Plio-Pleistocene environment, Lovejoy assumed that early hominids traveled between food sources, much as savanna baboons do. He also assumed that hominid females would have had fewer accidents and been less exposed to predators if they had refrained from moving too often. Lovejoy therefore speculated that males foraged farther afield for food and left the supposedly safer central area to the females and young.

Where does all-important bipedalism fit in? Nature favored males who were bipedal, because they could gather food and carry it back to their females and young. Thus, man the gatherer increased his number of living offspring. The problem with Lovejoy's hypothesis is that there is little or no comparative primate or ethnographic evidence to support its basic assumptions. If you see similarities with the man-the-hunter model, you are right. Either way, it is "man the provider." (As Zihlman points out, Lovejoy co-opted the male-gathering hypothesis from the earlier female-gathering hypothesis and even suggested that carrying devices might have been the first tools.[17])

Sex

What were the females doing when the males were away! Well, they were being faithful. As Lovejoy sees it, early hominids adopted our Western cultural tradition of monogamy. That way, a male could go away during the day and still be sure that it was he who had fathered his children. But wait, there's more to this male fantasy. Lovejoy believes that early hominid females were like modern women in several respects. Unlike many nonhuman primates, hominid women did not have specific periods in which they were in heat and mated (i.e., they did not go into estrus). Nor could males determine by visual inspection if a hominid woman was ovulating and therefore fertile. Therefore, copulatory vigilance was required to assure perpetuation of the species and reinforce the pair-bonds of couples. Early women obliged because, like contemporary human females, they were continually sexually receptive. (Now *there's* a fantasy.)

Needless to say, Lovejoy's theory did not receive positive critical acclaim from certain anthropologists, as shown by Zihlman's comment about Footnote 79 of Lovejoy's article:

> Lest there be any question about the chauvinistic undertones of Lovejoy's prehistoric family portrait, there is the coy reference, with regard to his assertion that females are perpetually sexually receptive, to a "personal communication" from his buddy, Donald C. Johanson, famous for his discovery of three-million-year-old "Lucy" and also well known for his Don Juan image. Lovejoy repeatedly invokes the "epigamic traits" (jargon for tits and ass) by which females succeed in attracting and holding their mates.[18]

For fun, the last word on bipedalism and the battle-of-the-sexes will be given to the late Nancy Tanner. Tanner's theory invokes the concept of sexual selection, an idea that goes back at least as far as Darwin. Features are sexually selected when they are preferred in one sex by the other and are passed down to future generations. A classic example is the beautiful tail feathers of male peacocks. Apparently, males have beautiful tails because females prefer to mate with (and, therefore, bear the offspring of) males who are so endowed. Tanner goes for woman the gatherer all the way:

> Among gathering mothers natural selection was strong for bipedalism: for walking from one forested area across grasslands to another, for freeing the hands for tool-use in obtaining food, for carrying babies and food . . .[19]

However, not to be sexist, Tanner allows males a role in the origins of bipedalism. Specifically, bipedal males were sexually selected by females:

> Whereas natural selection was more pertinent for bipedalism among gathering mothers, sexual selection was more significant for male bipedalism since their penises (especially when "upright") could be noted more readily when they walked bipedally.[19]

Tanner adds:

> As Freud long ago noted, an erect, unclothed male with an erect and quite visible penis might have proven noticeable and attractive.[19]

In this context, Jane Goodall's observation of a male chimpanzee named Shadow is interesting. Shadow was attacked by the females he courted until he invented an extraordinary courtship display that combined a bipedal stance, erect penis, and direct gaze. According to Goodall, Shadow's display worked wonders.[20]

Tanner's theory regarding sexual selection of bipedalism in male early hominids may seem frivolous, or even humorous. Nevertheless, it is noteworthy that relative to other primates, human males have enlarged penises.[21] Such "flasher" theories have also

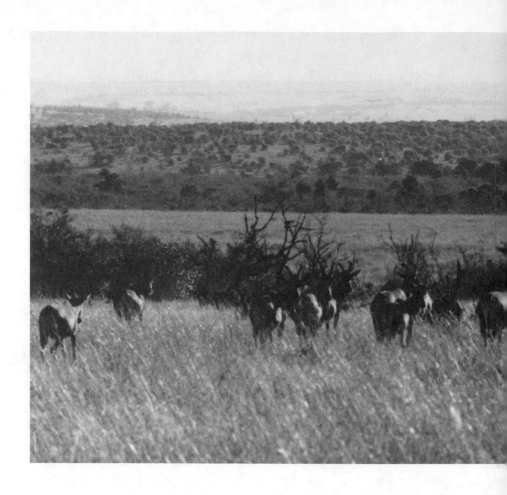

been applied to the large breasts of human women, as opposed to their relatively unendowed nonhuman primate cousins.

Wheeler's Explanation: Hominids Had It Made in the Shade

While all this hullabaloo was going on, a British biologist named Pete Wheeler of Liverpool Polytechnic sat back and quietly thought about the physiological factors involved with the shift to bipedalism. At the time early hominids were presumably becoming bipedal, the climate was getting drier. As a result, grassy savannas and woodlands replaced closed forests. Because food was

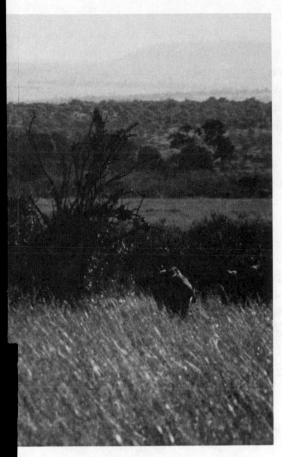

Early hominids had to travel through open country to find patches of food scattered within the mosaic environment. They may also have followed the seasonal migrations of savanna game. (Photograph by Dean Falk)

no longer uniformly distributed within forested habitats, it was harder to find. Thus, early hominids had to travel through open country to find patches of food scattered within the mosaic environment. They may also have followed the seasonal migrations of savanna game (meat on the hoof), as recently suggested by Mary Leakey and her colleagues.[22] Thus, there is no reason to rule out either plant or animal foods in the diets of early hominids. What's important is that hominids of both sexes traversed open spaces to feed. In so doing, they encountered intense solar radiation. *That* is the key to Wheeler's theory.[23]

Sunshine. As any dermatologist will attest, too much can be harmful to the skin. Further, if core body temperature increases even a moderate amount, heatstroke can result and cause brain

95

damage. Quadrupedal savanna mammals, like antelopes, have fur that protects their skin from solar radiation. They also have a special net of veins within the skull that prevents their brains from overheating. However, even with these adaptations, savanna animals take to the shade during the heat of day. (This was brought home to me on a recent train ride through Safari Park in San Diego. It was in the middle of a very hot day and, as our guide predicted, the animals we wished to see were all resting in the shade of trees.)

But humans have neither the marvelous net of veins nor the protection of overall body fur. How, then, did early hominids keep cool as they traveled out in the open, or scavenged and foraged for food without competition from other animals in the noonday sun? Wheeler has an eloquent and simple answer that is so obvious that others have overlooked it: Like pygmy chimpanzees, the CA was probably capable of a certain amount of bipedal locomotion or was preadapted for bipedalism. Early hominids were therefore able to minimize the amount of body surface that was directly exposed to solar radiation by walking bipedally. That way, only the shoulders and top of the head took a direct beating of rays when the sun was high in the sky. Put another way, early hominids created their own shade and were able to go about their business while they were at it.

Other adaptations also helped early hominids cope with thermal stress. With the shift to bipedalism, a coat of fur was no longer needed to protect the skin from direct solar radiation—except, that is, on top of the head and shoulders. In keeping with this, hair was retained on the head, but lost on large areas of the body. Hominid skin thus became (largely) naked. Especially efficient sweat glands also evolved as a means of cooling the recently denuded skin. (We humans are sweaty beasts, indeed, with the greatest sweating capacity for a given surface area of any known animal.)

A naked skin and associated cutaneous sweat glands allowed increased evaporation and, therefore, whole-body cooling in early hominids. According to Wheeler, such whole-body cooling helped prevent heatstroke and thereby released a physiological

refreshing departure, Richards has questioned the cliché that bipedalism led to freeing of the hands. He points out that chimpanzees use their feet like hands and that the tree-living common ancestor of humans and chimpanzees was probably also "four-handed." That means the transition to ground living was more likely to have enslaved the feet than to have freed the hands. If we accept the thesis that the foot became enslaved as a result of bipedalism, what of the hand? Did it not become liberated as a result of bipedalism (and able to fulfill itself by becoming skillful)? Maybe not. According to Richards:

> On becoming terrestrial the hand was never then "freed" from branch-holding, it brought the branch with it, as innumerable artist's impressions testify, along with the appropriate co-ordination schema. . . . It could be argued that even now many of us find a freed hand uncomfortable, feeling far more at ease holding something, be it a cigarette, a glass, a pen, a walking stick, the lapel of a jacket, something in our pocket, worry-beads, a necklace, or a stray lock of hair. Indeed we seem to be happiest with one hand, at least, engaged in gripping behavior, even after more than four million years . . .[26]

Whence the Fossils?

The above portrait of our earliest bipedal ancestor is gleaned from studies of comparative primate anatomy, molecular genetics, behavioral primatology, and the Laetoli footprints. But something is missing. Where are the fossilized skulls and teeth and long bones of early hominids? Unfortunately, except for a few jaws and teeth at Laetoli and one or two bits and pieces else-

Opposite page: In one of the few attempts to approach the question of the origin of bipedalism scientifically, biologist Pete Wheeler used this model (appropriately named "Boris") to quantify the relationship between posture and the amount of radiant heat load absorbed by the body. (Courtesy of Pete Wheeler)

where, the time between 5 and 3.2 million years ago is characterized by a gap in the hominid fossil record.[27] As we have seen, however, the tone of advocacy that was established when Raymond Dart first discovered australopithecines lives on and thrives. A mere lack of fossils does not prevent controversy and passion from governing discussions about how the CA looked and moved, or whether bipedalism was preferred more by males or females. The battle of the sexes over the evolution of bipedalism is entertaining, if a little silly. When it comes to the question of sex differences in the brain, however, we find ourselves on firmer ground.

on. However, in normal brains, this contralateral organization is far from complete because an additional 200 million nerve fibers cross directly between the two hemispheres, so that each is informed of what the other is doing. Besides facilitating communication between the two halves of the brain, these fibers allow the cerebral cortex to coordinate motor activities of both sides of the body. Thus, in brains of healthy individuals, both hemispheres get a total picture of what is going on. Not so for commissurotomy patients. Because surgery had permanently divided their brains, the cross talk that normally occurs between the two hemispheres is prevented. As a consequence, the left hemisphere sees things in the right but not the left half of the visual field, and perceives and manipulates objects that are held with the right but not the left hand. The converse is true for the right hemisphere. Furthermore, the functions of the right hemisphere are cut off (literally) from the main language areas that in most people are located in the left hemisphere.

Remarkably, commissurotomy patients seem unaware of their deficits, and appear to the casual observer to be normal. Apparently, during day-to-day activities, these patients unconsciously compensate for their disconnected hemispheres by cuing both hemispheres through speaking (which sends information into both ears), turning their heads (shifting visual fields), and touching or manipulating objects with both hands. As Sperry puts it,

> Normal behavior under ordinary conditions is favored also by many other unifying factors. Some of these are very obvious, like the fact that these two separate mental spheres have only one body and therefore they always get dragged to the same places, meet the same people, see and do the same things all the time and hence are bound to have a great overlap of common, almost identical experience.[2]

Nevertheless, Sperry was able to do controlled lateralized testing of commissurotomy patients by using procedures such as keeping the subject's hands isolated from each other and hidden from the subject's view, and projecting images exclusively into one visual field (with an instrument known as a tachistoscope). And, oh, what wonders his tests unraveled!

Under strict testing conditions, split-brain patients show themselves to be, literally, of two minds. Each hemisphere appears to experience its own separate consciousness and seems unaware of the mental events that occupy its other half. For example, if an object is placed in a patient's concealed left hand, she will not be able to *say* what it is, because speaking is a left-hemisphere function and that hemisphere receives input from the right hand, but not the left. Although the patient will report that she hasn't the foggiest idea of what she has just held in her left hand, her right hemisphere will then be able to select the correct object (with her left hand) from a number of choices. Similarly, objects placed in the right hand will be identified verbally or selected later from a group of objects by the right but not the left hand. Furthermore, both hemispheres can go about their respective endeavors simultaneously and cheerfully oblivious to each other. Thus, commissurotomy patients are very good at doing two things at once, as long as those two things are done by opposite hemispheres.

Prior to the research on split-brain patients, the right hemisphere was viewed as "an automaton lacking in conscious awareness."[3] This poor image held sway largely because of the left hemisphere's superiority for language. One of Sperry's most important findings was that the right hemisphere was not of such minor significance after all. It mentally outperformed the left hemisphere in a series of nonverbal, often spatial, tests, including (among others) the copying of designs, discrimination of shapes by both touch and sight, intuitively understanding geometrical properties, and reading faces. Careful testing also revealed that the right hemispheres of commissurotomy patients expressed emotions and possessed a sense of self that was as conscious and strong as that shown by their left hemispheres.

Over two decades later, Sperry's findings have been confirmed and widened by investigators using a variety of sophisticated techniques on enormous numbers of normal, as well as clinical, populations of humans. Methods for detecting brain asymmetries have included clinical research on brain-damaged individuals and patients in whom one hemisphere has been momentarily paralyzed by injection of a chemical (sodium amytal) into its blood supply. Lateralization studies have been carried out for sensory (e.g., discriminating how many points are touching an area of skin) and motor (handedness) activities. Normal individuals have been the subjects for numerous tachistoscopic visual and two-eared (dichotic) listening tests. In addition, basic anatomical asymmetries have been observed for certain brain structures. Finally, physiological correlates of brain lateralization have recently been obtained using a variety of techniques, among them electroencephalograms (EEG), the method of evoked potentials (EP), neuromagnetometry, and positron emission tomography (PET).[4]

The contemporary literature on brain lateralization is multifaceted and frequently difficult to interpret. Functional differences between the hemispheres are often subtle but statistically significant. Upon close inspection, however, contradictory results obtained by separate studies may often be attributed to slightly different methodologies or to differences in the populations investigated. For example, left-handers and the musically sophisticated do not test like the general population on some measures of brain asymmetry. Fortunately, certain generalizations about the left and right hemispheres float to the top, despite various complexities that plague this burgeoning field.

With these caveats in mind (and remembering that there are many exceptions), the following generalizations characterize the cerebral hemispheres of humans:[5] The left hemisphere is associated with language functions, skilled movements (e.g., like those engaged in by over 90 percent of right hands), and analytical, time-sequencing processes. This hemisphere is also involved in processing positive emotions. The right hemisphere, on the other hand, engages in global, holistic pursuits. Its visuospatial and mental imaging skills are superb, and it is also associated with musical abilities. Although the right hemisphere counterbalances the cheerful left hemisphere by processing negative emotions, it

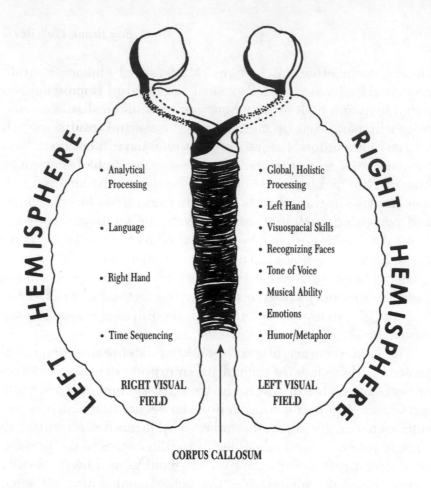

LEFT HEMISPHERE

RIGHT HEMISPHERE

- Analytical Processing
- Language
- Right Hand
- Time Sequencing

- Global, Holistic Processing
- Left Hand
- Visuospacial Skills
- Recognizing Faces
- Tone of Voice
- Musical Ability
- Emotions
- Humor/Metaphor

RIGHT VISUAL FIELD

LEFT VISUAL FIELD

CORPUS CALLOSUM

General specializations of left and right hemispheres. Top view of the brain (shown connected by the corpus callosum).

has a noticeably greater role than the left hemisphere in generally expressing emotions, as well as in reading them in others. In fact, although it is the left hemisphere that speaks, it is the right hemisphere that provides tone of voice, an important and sometimes decisive aspect of verbal communication. The right hemisphere also seems to have an edge over the left in recognizing faces, in certain aspects of humor, and in the ability to understand metaphor.

There are hints that certain biological substrates underlie functional lateralization of the two hemispheres. These substrates include asymmetries in the distribution of neurotransmitters that facilitate neurological activity, such as greater representation of norepinephrine in the right hemisphere and of dopamine (apparently involved with complex motor functions) in the left. Neurochemical asymmetries, in turn, may be the result of developmental (including intrauterine) events. Along these lines, limited evidence suggests that, prenatally, the right hemisphere matures more quickly than the left. If so, the two hemispheres will be exposed to slightly different intrauterine chemical environments at equivalent levels of maturity. Therein lies a key.[6]

The Mind-Body Problem Revisited

What is the relationship between conscious awareness and the brain? Although philosophers have been kicking the mind-body problem around for centuries, the new insights provided by commissurotomy studies have only recently become available. As noted above, a few contemporary workers infer from split-brain studies that each hemisphere has a separate mind of its own. Part of the reasoning underlying this conclusion is based on conflicting answers provided by the right and left hemispheres of individual patients in response to the same questions.[7] An interesting example of this doubling of consciousness was reported by commissurotomy patient N. V. J., who had been shopping with his wife:

> He was sitting next to her in the car as she was driving home. Between them was a large bag of groceries. He recounted, "My left hand reached into the bag and pulled out the licorice she had purchased for herself." I asked him, "Well, what's the matter with that?" He said, "I don't like licorice." I said, "Well, that is strange—what happened?" He said, "I ate it—but I didn't like it."[8]

Another example of interhemispheric competition occurred in the day-to-day routine of a female patient who experienced dramatic conflicts for several years following her surgery:

I open the closet door. I know what I want to wear. As I reach for something with my right hand, my left comes up and takes something different. I can't put it down if it's in my left hand. I have to call my daughter.[9]

Although my corpus callosum is intact and I frequently experience terrible dilemmas over what to wear, I am skeptical regarding the extreme view, held by some, that otherwise normal individuals have two separate minds in their heads. So, too, is Sperry (although he has been misquoted on the subject), who points out that even the question of whether there exists a right-left division of conscious experience in bisected brains is subject to debate.[10] According to Sperry, certain aspects of consciousness are *not* divided in split-brain patients. For example, sensations from both sides of the face and sounds experienced by both ears are represented in the two hemispheres. The same is true for sensations of crude pain, temperature, position sense, pressure, and visceral sensations like hunger. Thus, each disconnected hemisphere shares a sense of the positions and movements of body parts, as well as an awareness of the surrounding environment. Add to this the cross cuing that occurs in nontest situations and you get one unified consciousness, even in commissurotomy patients.

In sum, three decades of research on brain lateralization has expanded our understanding about asymmetrical representations of certain complementary cognitive abilities in the right and left hemispheres of human brains. No more and no less. Philosophers (and sometimes neuroscientists) too often lose sight of the fact that the two hemispheres are widely interconnected and that they function as a unit in normal brains. These investigators also continue to give undeserved priority to the left hemisphere and its language functions in discussions about what makes us truly human or conscious. (Musically naive as I am, I can have a dandy conscious experience that relies neither on language nor, in all probability, on other left-hemisphere functions by simply listening to classical music.[11]) As to the mind-body problem, Sperry defines consciousness as "a holistic or emergent, functional property of high-order brain activity."[12] And that's about as elegant a definition as one can hope for.

Different Sexes, Different Brains

As populations, males and females test differently for certain abilities that are neurologically lateralized. Some workers have questioned the utility of studying such differences because there is usually massive overlap in the distributions of these traits for the two sexes. In these cases, numerous individuals of the weaker sex (for some tasks it is males; for others, females) outperform many of the stronger sex. Despite the fact that sex differences are frequently small, they are often real (i.e., statistically significant). Furthermore, the sex differences that have been detected form a fascinating pattern that provides clues about the evolution of brain lateralization.

Females tend to outperform males slightly but significantly on tests of verbal abilities, including reading comprehension, essay writing, anagrams, and (especially) measures of spoken language.[13] Interestingly, females appear to be more left-hemisphere biased for general motor expression than males, as shown by their greater rightward skill for fine motor tasks such as finger-tapping and cursive writing. Compared with males, females are also subtly biased for certain emotional skills such as understanding nonverbal body language (this may, in fact, be one basis for good old women's intuition).

Males, on the other hand, test better than females for perception and manipulation of spatial relationships, such as mental rotation of figures, maze tracing, map reading, rod-and-frame alignment tests, and remembering positions of numbers. They are also better at left-right discriminations, disembedding figures, and localizing points. As is well known, males outperform females in certain areas of mathematics, particularly on calculus and geometry problems.[14] Finally, there is some indication that males also excel at musical abilities such as composition.[15] This raises the interesting possibility that the manipulation of auditory space involved in musical composition is based on cognitive processes that are similar to those that underlie another right-hemisphere activity at which males excel, namely perception and rotation of visual shapes. This seems plausible because music, like visual images, has contours and corners.

The above generalizations are gleaned from many hundreds of studies across a diverse spectrum of human activities based on musical, visuospatial, auditory, motor, emotional, and linguistic skills. Despite the complexity, confusion, and related political issues that abound in the literature, this body of information converges on a clear bottom line: Finely-shaded but significant sex differences characterized human behaviors. And of all those differences, the largest (no fine shading here) is the one in which males are favored for certain visuospatial skills such as the mental folding task illustrated below.[16] The fact that males are particularly good at getting around—reading maps, tracing mazes, and mentally manipulating spatial arrangements in visual and auditory modes—should not be viewed as in any way detracting from females. I believe that these skills contributed to the remarkable evolution of our species—in both sexes.

Males have somewhat larger brains than females, but this may simply reflect their generally larger body size. Beyond this, specific anatomical differences have been reported for the brains of men and women in several regions including the massa intermedia, planum temporal, anterior commissure, corpus callosum, and two nuclei of the anterior hypothalamus.[17] There is also some evidence that the *pattern* of brain lateralization differs for the two sexes. According to one survey of the literature, females seem to process certain kinds of information with both hemispheres, whereas males tend to rely more on one hemisphere or the other.[18] For example, the incidence of aphasia (an inability to use or understand words) after left-hemisphere lesions is at least three times higher in men than in women. This suggests that females may process language more with both hemispheres.

However, the generalization that males are more lateralized than females needs to be tempered with findings from studies by

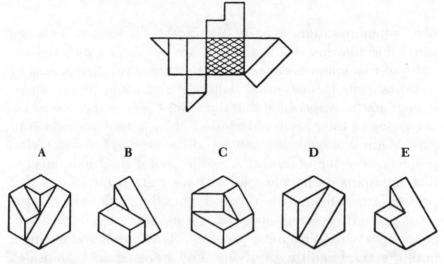

A B C D E

Certain spatial aptitudes seem to be (on average) better developed in males than in females. Select the appropriate figure that represents what the upper figure would look like when it is folded into a three-dimensional object (the shaded portion is the bottom). See note 16, chapter 5 for answer. (Figure courtesy Roland Guay)

Doreen Kimura of the University of Western Ontario, in Canada. She found that speech disorders and manual difficulties occurred significantly more often in women because of damage to the left frontal lobe, whereas these conditions were caused more often in men by damage to their left posterior parietal and temporal lobes. Kimura concluded that for women (who have stronger tendencies toward right-handedness than men), manual skills are at least as dependent as speech on the left frontal lobe. Thus, women may be more asymmetrical for frontal lobe motor activities, and men for functions that are subserved by more posterior regions of the brain. If so, the sexes appear to differ in the front-to-back organization within hemispheres, as well as the right-left pattern for the whole brain.[19]

There is less clinical information available about the degree to which visuospatial skills are lateralized in the sexes. However, a small number of studies do show that males are more dependent on their right hemispheres for certain visuospatial tasks. Investigations of the patterns of hemispheric blood flow during tasks like mental rotation indicate significant differences between males and females. These findings are consistent with the hypothesis that males are specialized for some visuospatial skills.

Certain neuroanatomical findings regarding brain shape strengthen the impression that the sexes differ in the overall organization of their brains. Marjorie LeMay, a radiologist at Harvard Medical School, has pioneered the study of asymmetrical projections of the brain that are called petalias. She discovered that right-handed people tend to have right frontal lobes that project farther than the left frontal lobes (i.e., a right frontal petalia) and left occipital lobes that extend more than their right counterparts (left occipital petalias). This configuration gives both the brain and the overlying skull a characteristic lopsided appearance that can be seen in CAT scans and x-rays. LeMay showed that left-handers are characterized by higher frequencies of the reverse conditions (namely, left frontal and right occipital petalias).

LeMay's research is very important because it demonstrates a statistical link between brain shape and handedness. Results of a recent study confirm LeMay's earlier findings. The latter study also shows that greater degrees of frontal and occipital asymmetries are present in men than in women. Furthermore, reversals of the typical petalia patterns are more common in women, even though their incidence of left-handedness is slightly less than that for men.[20]

Sex Hormone Research

Quickly recite the tongue twister "a box of mixed biscuits in a biscuit mixer" five times! Not exactly a piece of cake, huh? Elizabeth Hampson, of the University of Western Ontario, and Doreen Kimura have recently shown that women are significantly better at this task when their monthly cycles are at peak estrogen and progesterone levels—just before ovulation and again during the last week before menstruation.[21] On the other hand, when estrogen and progesterone levels are low, during and right after menstruation, the same women do not do as well on this test or on other measures of speeded motor coordination like finger-tapping or peg-assembly tasks. Since women generally outper-form men on tests of skilled motor coordination, it appears that high estrogen and progesterone levels enhance female skills.

But what effect do female sex hormones have on the visuospa-tial tasks at which males usually excel? In another part of the same study, each woman was given a rod-and-frame test, at two care-fully selected times during her cycle. (The goal of the test is to align a rod to the true vertical against a deceptively tilted back-ground, and males are generally better at it than females.) The results were striking. The subjects were significantly less accu-rate at aligning the rod at the midluteal phase of their cycles, when estrogen and progesterone levels were high, than during menstruation, when they were low.

As the foregoing discussion shows, visuospatial skills (at which men usually excel) are enhanced in menstruating women, just when their generally superior motor skills are inhibited. Hamp-son and Kimura therefore conclude that women's performances on cognitive tasks are influenced by their fluctuating hormonal states. They also suggest that sex differences on these and other cognitive tests may have a substantial hormonal basis. For exam-ple, the neurotransmitter dopamine plays a role in motor coordi-nation, and it is possible that sex hormones influence its release in the brain.

A key to sex differences in performance on cognitive tests may lie in the prenatal environment. Sheri Berenbaum, of Chicago Medical School, and Melissa Hines, from the University of Cali-fornia at Los Angeles, studied play behavior in children with con-genital adrenal hyperplasia (CAH), a genetic disorder that causes an individual to release excessive amounts of androgen (a male hormone) before and after birth.[22] They found that compared with their normal sisters, CAH girls played significantly more often with boys' toys than with girls' toys. (Normal children have sexually specific toy preferences. Boys like to play with vehicles and building toys, while girls prefer kitchens and dolls.) It there-fore appears that sex differences in cognition (in this case, play behavior) are at least partially hormonally primed, and this priming takes place at early stages of development.

Hines summarizes other evidence for hormonal influences on sex differences in human cognition and notes further that exposure to low levels of hormones during development is always associated with reduction in male-typical cognitive traits, whereas exposure to high levels of hormones increases these traits:

> First, adolescent girls and young women exposed to excess testosterone and other androgens prenatally, because they have a genetic defect called congenital adrenal hyperplasia (CAH), have been reported to show enhanced performance on measures of visuospatial abilities. Second, men exposed to lower than normal levels of androgen from early life, because they have idiopathic hypogonadotrophic hypogonadism, have been found to show reduced visuospatial abilities. Third, women exposed to higher than normal levels of estrogen prenatally, because their mothers were prescribed the synthetic estrogen, diethylstilbestrol (DES), during pregnancy, have been found to show increased language lateralization. Finally, girls and women exposed to lower than normal levels of hormones, because of prenatal ovarian regression associated with the genetic disorder of Turner syndrome, have reduced visuospatial abilities and reduced language lateralization.[23]

Albert Galaburda, of Harvard Medical School, and the late Norman Geschwind have developed a rather speculative, but interesting, theory about brain lateralization that is based on prenatal priming of the nervous system with sex hormones. Their reasoning goes something like this: There is some evidence that the cerebral convolutions of fetuses develop earlier on the surfaces of their right, rather than their left, hemispheres. Therefore, some influence probably slows growth of parts of the left hemisphere. In those individuals for whom left-hemisphere growth is particularly slowed, corresponding parts of the right hemisphere compensate by growing faster and possibly larger.

This results in especially well-developed right-hemisphere visuospatial functions and a relatively high incidence of left-handedness. On the other hand, left-hemisphere functions suffer from being left behind, as is indicated by higher incidences of language disorders such as dyslexia or stuttering.

As it turns out, the configuration of both positive and negative traits that are said to be associated with slowed growth of the left hemisphere is manifested much more in males than in females. Galaburda and Geschwind therefore conclude that the influence that theoretically slows growth of the left hemisphere is probably male-related, and they offer the male hormone testosterone as a likely candidate because developing males are exposed to much greater quantities of it than are developing females. Thus, brain lateralization and the priming related to sex differences in cognitive abilities may both be mediated by the action of testosterone on the cerebral cortex, especially during the third month of intra-uterine life.[24]

Theories such as this are built largely, but not exclusively, on animal models. This is because, for ethical reasons, scientists are very limited in the experiments that can be performed on people. In order to study questions about brain evolution and lateralization, my colleagues from Washington University in St. Louis and I recently analyzed endocasts that were prepared from hundreds of skulls from one of the most widely used animal models in medical research, the rhesus monkey. These endocasts were from known individuals of certain age and sex, and they revealed many details about skull sutures, cortical sulci, and brain shape. Two of our findings are of interest with respect to Galaburda and Geschwind's hypothesis.[25]

First, during postnatal development in monkeys, some cranial sutures closed significantly sooner on the right than on the left side, but never the reverse. Recall that the convolutions of human fetal brains tend to develop on the right side first. If an asymmetry in skull growth like that seen in monkeys also occurs in humans (a reasonable hypothesis), then there may be a *general developmental gradient*, whereby the right side of the cranium and its contents are slightly outpacing the growth of the left side.

Our second finding was a dramatic sex difference in the age at which adult brain size (estimated from cranial capacity) was reached in rhesus monkeys. Females attained their adult sizes by about four years of age, whereas males did not achieve their adult brain sizes until they were six years old. If a similar pattern also characterizes human brain growth, it could help explain why males appear more lateralized than females (in some respects), without necessarily having to argue that testosterone inhibits left-hemisphere growth. To wit: If right hemispheres are pro-grammed to develop at slightly faster rates than left hemispheres in both sexes, and if brain growth continues longer in males, then the two hemispheres of males will grow farther apart (i.e., be-come more asymmetrical) than those of females. This hypothesis, brought to you courtesy of the standard rhesus monkey animal model, seems well worth exploring.

Despite an ongoing revolution in the neurosciences, the human brain remains, in many respects, a little black box that can only be pondered from the outside. However, the few glimpses we get of the brain's inner workings do gel into three useful in-sights: First, sex hormones play an important role during the brain's development, and they subsequently influence cognition. Second, the interaction of the prenatal chemical environment with the *timing* of specific neurological developments is of defin-itive importance for the brain's structure and, therefore, its even-tual functions. Finally, the brains of males and females are to some extent organized differently.

So which influences brain development, nature or nurture? The answer, of course, is both. Are the small but significant dif-ferences between males and females due to genes or cultural fac-tors? Again, both factors are important. Although brain lateralization is undoubtedly rooted in a genetic substrate, it is important to keep in mind that traits selected for in one sex are usually automatically increased in the other sex. (This is due to the way genes mix and match as they are passed from parents to offspring of both sexes.)

At least one pioneer in the study of sex hormones and behavior is well aware of the importance of cultural factors (including sexism) for determining behavior. Noting that women outperform men on verbal and dexterity skills, Estelle Ramey, professor emeritus at Georgetown University, says: "So what do [men] say about women? That they talk too much. Even when you have the advantage, you can't win." Such biases are engendered by women as well, she adds. "Females also have the advantage in digital dexterity. So do they become neurosurgeons? No, they do needlepoint! In other words, the biology is just the barest beginning."[26]

Brain Lateralization in Other Animals

Philosophers tend to exaggerate the extent to which *Homo sapiens* is special and set apart from other animals. Until fairly recently, such anthropocentrism characterized the thinking about brain lateralization. Consequently, it took many years for workers to accept the idea that other animals have lateralized brains—especially since this fact seems to be contradicted by a lack of language and right-handedness in nonhuman species. But lateralized brains they have. Today, asymmetrical nervous systems have been found in a wide variety of animals that range from rodents to birds to primates.

The unfolding of this information is one of those rare scientific success stories that I love. It began with research in the early 1970s, when Stanley Glick made two serendipitous observations about rats. Glick, who now chairs the Department of Pharmacology and Toxicology at Albany Medical Center, first found that drugging trained rats with amphetamine increases their side preferences in pressing levers. He then discovered that amphetamine induces more circling behavior in untrained rats. (Though they do so less intensely, normal undrugged rats rotate at night, in the same direction induced by amphetamine.) At the time of Glick's observations, it was known that vigorous circling could also be induced in rats by lesions to deep parts of one side of the brain that damaged neurons containing dopamine. Glick therefore postulated that amphetamine caused his rats to prefer one side in

117

lever pressing or rotation because of its action on an asymmetrical dopaminergic system.

In a 1974 report in *Science,* Betty Zimmerberg (currently at Williams College) and her colleagues actually demonstrated the existence of an asymmetrical dopaminergic system in normal rats. And the concentration of dopamine turned out to be significantly higher on the nonpreferred side. Together, Zimmerberg and Glick concluded that these and other results indicated that circling is a stereotyped spatial behavior that derives from a deep neuroanatomical asymmetry. This means that rats have lateralized nervous systems that are responsible for their lateralized circling. Curiously, male and female rats have a slight tendency to circle in opposite directions.

How did scientists respond to these dramatic findings? "At first, people didn't believe us," says Glick. "Then, when they finally did believe the results, they said 'So what? They're only rats, not people.'" There was only one thing to do. In 1982, Glick and his colleagues investigated the distribution of a variety of neurotransmitters, including dopamine, in human brains. Not only did they find an asymmetry in the distribution of dopamine in these brains, it turned out to be twice as high as that for rats. Just as dopamine levels were higher on the side opposite circling preference in rats, dopamine levels of humans were higher on the side opposite the most frequently preferred hand.

But circling behavior is one thing, and handedness is another. Or is it? What about rotation in humans? Do people turn in preferred directions like rats? If so, do males and females also prefer opposite directions? Eager to answer these questions, Glick and a colleague designed an electronic rotometer that humans could wear on a belt. This device measured exactly the same kinds of rotational movements that had been observed in rats. Although they had no idea of the kind of counts obtained by the device, seventy-four male and sixty-one female students, physicians, and hospital employees agreed to wear the rotometer for seven to eight consecutive hours. People proved to be just like rats! Without realizing it, most of the men and women preferentially rotated to the left or to the right during a routine day. (You probably

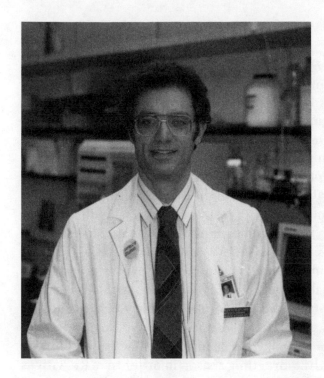

Stanley Glick. "At first people didn't believe us. Then, when they finally did believe the results, they said 'so what? they're only rats, not people.'" Glick's pioneering work was instrumental in establishing that brain lateralization is typical of many animals, not just humans.

do too.) As in rats, female humans rotated more than males, and the sexes also differed with respect to their overall directional preferences. Left-hemisphere-dominant men rotated more to the right, whereas left-hemisphere-dominant women rotated more to the left.

Because of Glick's research, investigators can no longer say "So what" to rats. Or to birds or primates, for that matter. Furthermore, a review of experimental studies for various mammals based on locomotor, neurochemical, lesion, and neuroanatomical measures shows that *gender* is a major determinant for patterns of behavioral and brain asymmetries. In fact, sex differences in locomotor asymmetries, such as circling in rodents, are the rule rather than the exception.[27]

An Evolutionary Model

Why did brain lateralization get started in the first place?[28] The work of Glick and his colleagues suggests that in the beginning

119

there may have been circling. But what good is that? Simply put, if one wanders off, one wanders back to the safety of the nest, if one is a rodent, or full circle back to the starting point, if one is a lost human explorer. At least for the rodent, finding the way home would presumably be an adaptive trait favored by natural selection. That is, homing rodents would have longer lives and leave more offspring than those unfortunates who get lost. I asked Glick what function he thought might be served by a preferred direction of rotation, and he suggested that rats who don't waste time deciding which way to turn might be better able to get away from attackers. This too would no doubt be adaptive.

But why the sex difference? A clue to this puzzle is provided by other rodents called voles. Voles look like small burrowing mice, and they come in two kinds. Prairie voles from the Midwest are monogamous, with both sexes sticking close to home. Meadow voles from Pennsylvania are polygynous, and males wander far afield during breeding season in order to mate with as many females as possible. The two species of voles are, therefore, perfect subjects for testing whether or not sex differences in visuospatial skills are associated with males getting about in the world and, if so, whether or not visuospatial skills contribute to breeding success. And that's just what Steven Gaulin and Randall FitzGerald, of the University of Pittsburgh, did in an intriguing set of experiments.[29]

During the first part of their study, Gaulin and FitzGerald trapped voles of both species and fitted them with small radio transmitters. After the voles were released, daily ranges and total ranges were determined from each subject's broadcasts. The results confirmed that male meadow voles expanded their ranges during the breeding season, whereas female meadow voles did not. In contrast, the monogamous prairie voles showed no sex differences, at any time, in their ranging patterns.

During the second part of the investigation, the voles of both species were retrapped and tested for visuospatial ability in laboratory mazes. In keeping with Gaulin and FitzGerald's earlier findings, only polygynous meadow voles showed consistent male superiority on the spatial tasks. It is therefore a good guess that visuospatial skills evolved in male meadow voles because their far-ranging search for mates contributed to their reproductive success (which, after all, is what evolution is all about).

But vision is not the only sense that is important for breeding success. Because of their habitats, arboreal species such as birds rely more on auditory senses. For example, canaries use songs to announce their presence to neighbors and to claim breeding territories. More important for our discussion, it is male songbirds who sing to attract mates. Further, birdsong is neurologically lateralized to left forebrain structures, which are three to four times larger in adult male canaries who sing complex songs than in adult females who sing simpler songs.[30] Apparently, birdsong contributes to reproductive success, and it is reasonable to conclude that sex differences in the behavior, as well as the neurological asymmetries underlying birdsong, were selected for in this context.

Unlike the bird and rodent examples, nonhuman primates rely heavily on both visual and vocal communication systems. And in humans, at least, the visual and vocal systems are generally lateralized to right and left hemispheres, respectively. Taking a cue from the evolution of other mammals, could sex differences in visuospatial and vocal communication skills have been selected for in the primate ancestors of early hominids?

Although this question is difficult to address, there is evidence that permits one to engage in educated speculation. Like humans, macaque monkeys are left-hemisphere dominant for processing socially meaningful vocalizations and right-hemisphere dominant for certain visual discriminations. Macaques also manifest petalia patterns and other cortical asymmetries that are similar to those of humans. These findings, along with a number of other recent studies, suggest that the substrate for human brain lateralization was present long ago—during *early* anthropoid evolution.[31]

A recent and surprising survey of handedness across the primate order also suggests that early anthropoids were neurologically lateralized. Peter MacNeilage, of the University of Texas at Austin, and his colleagues showed that nonhuman primates tend to be left-handed when reaching for food and right-handed for manipulative tasks. According to MacNeilage's evolutionary scenario, the initial primate adaptation (indicated by studies on prosimians) involved right-hemisphere specialization for visually guided reaching with the left hand. Subsequently, the left hemisphere of higher (anthropoid) primates became specialized for right-hand manipulation and bimanual coordination. This model, therefore, gives primacy to specialization of the right hemisphere for visuospatial functions during early primate evolution.

From the above, we may conclude that anthropoid primates indeed have lateralized brains and that this trait probably enjoyed a long evolutionary history. Of all the anthropoids, of course, *Homo sapiens* is the most lateralized. Since gender is a determinant for patterns of behavioral and brain asymmetries in mammals including humans, we may speculate that gender was probably an important factor in the development of brain lateralization in ancestral primates. The fossil and archaeological record suggests that by two million years ago, early *Homo* had brains that were lateralized along the lines of our own. Meanwhile, we are left wondering about sex differences in patterns of brain lateralization in early hominids.

Unfortunately, attention to gender is often missing from studies of hominid brain evolution. The knapping (shaping) of stone tools requires special visuospatial skills, and it would be interesting to know the sex distribution of early knappers. Were they predominantly male? As spatial competence increased during the evolution of tool production (beautifully described by Thomas Wynn[32]), were sex differences in patterns of behavioral and brain asymmetries also evolving?

I have an image of one of our distant mammalian ancestors who lived over sixty-five million years ago. The ancestor is male and it is mating season. He's good at spatial navigation and temporarily extends his daily range in search of mates. Because of a good cognitive map, he is able to return home later and to repeat the process during the next mating season. During his life, he fathers many offspring.

Thanks to Wynn, I also have an image of one of the mammal's distant, future descendants. It is a knapper making a bifacial stone tool, some 300,000 years ago. As the tool takes shape, the knapper uses notions of perspective, the control of spatial quantity, and an understanding of composition. Overall shape is very important to the knapper. When it is finished, the tool has a regular cross section. It is gorgeous. And all because the knapper's distant ancestor was good at getting around and delivered the genes for skilled visuospatial abilities to his offspring. The knapper is satisfied with the way the tool has turned out. She packs up and goes home.[33]

Despite my cheerful image of woman-the-knapper, the previous discussion of bipedalism and the battle of the sexes shows that the role women played during human evolution is a subject of much recent debate. Nevertheless, this discourse represents an improvement over the old unquestioned assumption that males were the primary focus of selection for various good and noble human features. And of all the ancestral females who have lived during the past five million years, one in particular has created havoc in the hominid fossil record. Her name is Lucy.

I would need the thick hide I had grown during the debate over the lunate sulcus, as well as everything I had learned about the politics of paleoanthropology, for my research related to that little lady.

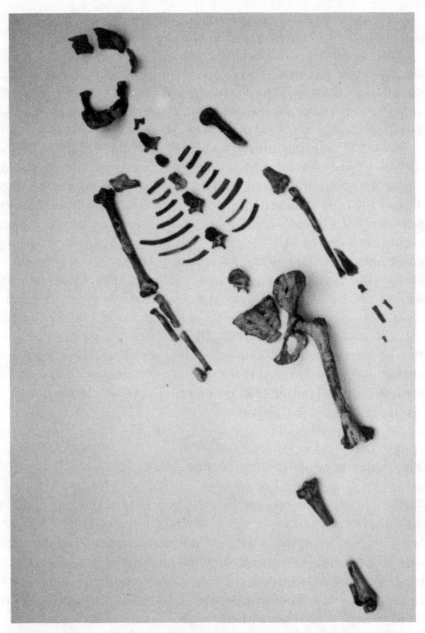

Lucy. Nearly 40 percent of her skeleton was discovered eroding from sand deposits in the Hadar region of the Afar Depression in Ethiopia. (Photograph by John Reader, copyright © 1992/Science Photo Library)

tain a cranial capacity or to provide other definitive clues about the identity of her species.

Although Lucy is the most famous fossil hominid from the Hadar site in Ethiopia, she is not the only one. She had lots of company, including the so-called "First Family" of thirteen individuals from one particular location. According to Johanson, this group of individuals lived together, and died together as a result of some natural catastrophe such as a flash flood.[1] He believed that they may even have been relatives. However, these individuals were extremely varied in their physical appearance and geological evidence suggests that they were fossilized and buried separately. In other words, these early hominids may not have constituted one group.

Although Lucy eventually became Johanson's claim to fame, he did not really know what to make of her at first. Which relative did she most resemble? Which species did she represent? Johanson's first assessment of Lucy was published (with Maurice Taieb) in 1976.[2] At that time, he thought she might be a primitive version of a gracile australopithecine. It is significant that Johanson also thought that three species of early hominids may have been represented at Hadar: gracile australopithecines, robust australopithecines, and early *Homo*.

The Naming of *Australopithecus afarensis*

At the time I was contemplating the contents of the Red Cave, a former classmate of mine was studying the early hominid fossils from the Hadar region and from Laetoli, Tanzania. His name was Tim White, and he was instrumental in convincing Johanson to lump all of the fossils from these two sites together into one new species, *Australopithecus afarensis*. This was quite a departure from Johanson's earlier assessment.

When White (now at the University of California, Berkeley) and I began our graduate studies at the University of Michigan, its physical anthropology program was known for supporting a "single-species hypothesis." According to this school of thought,

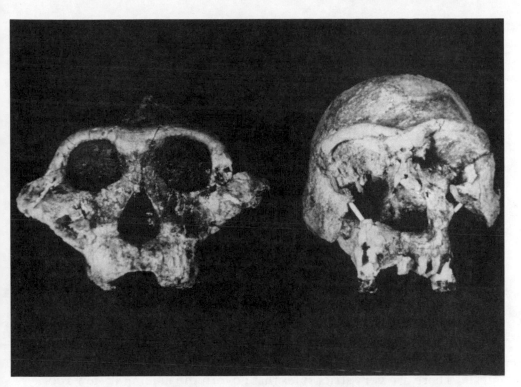

With the discovery of ER 406, a robust australopithecine (left), and ER 3733, a contemporaneous early Homo erectus *specimen (right), the single-species hypothesis lost its luster. (Photograph by R. E. Leakey, copyright National Museums of Kenya)*

there was only one species of early hominid living at any given time; therefore, two species of australopithecines had never coexisted. Thus, the variation seen in australopithecines was attributed to sex, rather than species, differences. Robust australopithecines were believed to be males and gracile australopithecines were supposedly females. We graduate students at Michigan were brought up on this hypothesis. And we believed it.

At least we did until 1976. That's when the single-species hypothesis died rather suddenly because of a fatal blow struck by a paper in *Nature* by Richard Leakey and Alan Walker. It was entitled *"Australopithecus, Homo erectus, and the single species hypothesis"* and revealed that two beautiful skulls coexisted in Kenya, some 1.5 million years ago. One was a robust australopithecine (KNM-ER 406), the other an early *Homo erectus*

(KNM-ER 3733).[3] Clearly the single-species hypothesis was no longer tenable.

However, with some justification, investigators continued to emphasize sex as an important source of variation in early hominids. For example, Johanson and his colleagues viewed the large fossils from Laetoli and Hadar as males and the smaller ones as females. They then proceeded to lump the fossils from both sites into one new species (*Australopithecus afarensis*). With the advantage of hindsight, this melding of fossils from two sites now seems questionable for several reasons: it is currently believed that, besides being in different countries, Laetoli and Hadar had different climates (Laetoli's was more arid), had different habitats (evergreen bushland at Hadar, open savanna vegetation at Laetoli),[4] and were separated by at least half a million years of time. Also, the fossils from Laetoli are relatively few and consist mostly of jaws, teeth, and footprints, while cranial fragments that are critical for assessing taxonomic status are mostly lacking.

There are very strict rules that govern the naming of new zoological species. These rules are formally spelled out in the *International Code of Zoological Nomenclature.*[5] According to the Code, new scientific names must be made readily accessible to the scientific community in a publication. If an investigator has something really important to communicate, he or she generally tries to publish in the best possible journal. And the best journals are peer reviewed. Articles submitted to these journals are either rejected or accepted for publication on the basis of anonymous reviews by a number of experts. Even if an article is rejected, the author usually benefits by receiving copies of the anonymous reviews that often contain suggestions for improving the manuscript. Sometimes editors will provisionally accept an article for publication (i.e., accept it on the condition that the author make certain revisions suggested by the reviewers).

The process of peer review is not a perfect one. But it does assure a certain amount of scientific give-and-take within disciplines, as well as the improvement of many manuscripts prior to their publication. Inferior articles get weeded out by the review process at peer-reviewed journals. Examples of peer-reviewed journals are the *American Journal of Physical Anthropology, Journal of Human Evolution, Science,* and *Nature.* Although the Code does not specify that new names must be published in peer-reviewed journals, any of the above would have been an appropriate forum in which to name a new species of early hominid. However, Johanson, White, and Coppens named *Australopithecus afarensis* in 1978 in *Kirtlandia,* which is described on its inside cover as "an occasional publication of The Cleveland Museum of Natural History." (In fairness, it is to their credit and the field's benefit that Johanson and his colleagues went on to publish full and detailed descriptions of the Hadar material in a 1982 issue of the *American Journal of Physical Anthropology.*)

More telling is the response of Johanson, White, and Coppens to Article 13a(i) of the Code, which requires that the published name be "accompanied by a statement that purports to give characters differentiating the taxon." Given White's education at Michigan, it is not surprising that the investigators attributed the variation in their species to strong sexual dimorphism. However, the *Kirtlandia* account of variation in so-called *Australopithecus afarensis* went further:

> The authors recognize that individual traits and even single specimens in the new collection can be matched in other samples representing different taxa (e.g., *Australopithecus africanus* Dart 1925, *Homo habilis* Leakey, Tobias and Napier 1964).[6]

In other words, *Australopithecus afarensis* was so variable that some of its specimens looked like gracile australopithecines, while others looked like *Homo habilis*!

Since the above was written, the Hadar dates have been reassessed, and it turns out that they are likely to have been contemporaneous with the gracile australopithecine site of Makapansgat, South Africa.[7] This raises a dilemma for the next discoverer of a fossil australopithecine from a previously undiscovered 3.2-million-year-old site. What species should it be assigned to if it is one of those specimens that matches both *Australopithecus africanus*

Dart and *Australopithecus afarensis*? Can two fossils that are identical (not to mention contemporaneous) reasonably be assigned to two different species? I do not believe so.

According to Johanson and White's preferred taxonomic scheme (published in *Science* in 1979), their new species was the *only* australopithecine on the line leading directly to *Homo sapiens*.[8] Everybody else's australopithecines were placed on a sidebranch that became extinct without issue. By now, the reader will not be surprised to learn that everybody else did not approve of Johanson and White's genealogy. In fact, neighbors (some of them named Leakey and Tobias and Walker[9]) began whispering suspicions that there might have been a mix-up at the hospital. But having named the new species and passed out the cigars, would the proud parents agree to a blood test?

The Evidence from Cranial Blood Flow

My reaction to all of this at the time? Mostly, I was amazed at the rapidity with which much of the field accepted the new species. Other than that, I was too busy defending my position on the position of the lunate sulcus to develop much of an opinion about the details of early hominid phylogeny. Then in 1982, quite by accident, I found myself immersed in blood.

Cranial remains of australopithecines and early *Homo* were my subject matter and, once again, I was spending my summer doing research in African museums. For the first time, I also saw numerous casts of the cranial remains from the Hadar early hominids. Although convolutions and sulci were my primary interest, that summer I became fascinated with a particular feature that showed up on some of the fossils. It had to do with cranial blood flow.

The feature that caught my attention was a dramatic groove located inside the back of the braincase. This large groove is called the occipital/marginal (or O/M) sinus, and it is rarely present in a form large enough to leave a groove in apes or living people. In life, the enlarged O/M sinus of early hominids provided a major pathway for draining blood from the skull. But only for *some* early hominids. What intrigued me was that all of the scorable robust australopithecines (there are now seven) and all of the scorable Hadar early hominids (five specimens) had this feature, while only one of (now) six gracile australopithecines showed it.[10] (That specimen was Taung, which may have been incorrectly placed with gracile instead of robust australopithecines because of its young age, as the reader will recall.) Contrary to Johanson and White's taxonomic scheme in which robust australopithecines and the Hadar early hominids were completely separated, presence of the unusual O/M sinus in all scorable members of both of these two groups suggested to me that they might, in fact, be directly related.

But why did some early hominids have an O/M sinus? What was its function? For that, I turned to my colleague and fellow paleontologist, Glenn Conroy, now in the Department of Anatomy and Neurobiology at Washington University School of Medicine. Glenn agreed that it seemed to be too much of a coincidence to find the highly unusual O/M sinus in all members of two different groups of unrelated early hominids. We decided to put our heads together about heads.

Glenn and I knew that Lucy and company were among the earliest known bipeds. That led us to wonder if the O/M sinus had something to do with the origins of bipedalism. As a starting point, we decided to find out whether or not there was a general relationship between posture and cranial blood flow in living people. Within weeks, we located and studied a number of relevant clinical and physiological reports that made it clear that cranial blood flow depends very much on posture. And not just for humans.

Monkeys, snakes, people, and giraffes are all subject to the constraints of gravity. In all of these animals, blood flow changes with a shift in body posture from a horizontal (lying down) to a vertical (standing up) position. (For snakes, blood flow differs between horizontal positions on the ground and vertical hanging postures in trees.) A major reason why blood flow changes with altered postures is because gravity places different stresses

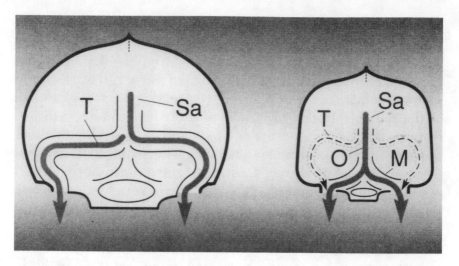

Blood flow routes that appear in the back of human skulls (left) and the Hadar hominids and robust australopithecines (right). Sa, superior sagittal sinus; T, transverse sinus; O, occipital sinus; and M, marginal sinus. In humans, cranial blood flows through the transverse sinuses and out of the skull. In the hominids on the right, blood flows straight down the O/M sinus before exiting the cranium.

(called hydrostatic pressures) on horizontal and vertical columns of fluid (such as blood in veins).

To understand this, imagine a long tube half-filled with water. If the tube is vertical, all of the water is in its bottom half. When the tube is completely tilted over on its side, however, the water is redistributed along its entire length. Now imagine that the tube contains little holes that are sparsely but evenly distributed over its entire surface. When the tube is vertical, the water drains out of the holes in its bottom. When it is horizontal, on the other hand, the water exits through holes all along the tube's side. To wit: Different postures, different exits for fluid. And all because of gravity.

Conroy and I learned that the same thing happens with blood that is draining from peoples' skulls. If an individual is lying down, cranial blood flows out through the internal jugular veins. When the person stands up, however, most of the exiting cranial blood shifts away from the jugulars and into a network of veins that surrounds the spinal cord. That network of veins is called the vertebral plexus. Our bipedal existence depends on it! We were on to something.

Our next task was to determine if there was a relationship between an enlarged O/M sinus and the vertebral plexus of veins. Again, we studied the literature and, again, the answer was affirmative. Most humans have small O/M sinuses (not big enough to leave grooves in skulls) and these usually have numerous connections with the vertebral plexus of veins. More to the point, in a study of one hundred human cadavers, nine had relatively large O/M sinuses.[11] Seven of these nine O/M sinuses were connected to the vertebral plexus of veins. Clearly, it was a good bet that the even larger O/M sinuses of early hominids were also connected with the vertebral plexus of veins. After all, if cranial blood flows to the vertebral plexus of veins when a person stands up, it makes sense that a route leading to the vertebral plexus would be enlarged in some of the earliest bipeds.

Conroy and I took our findings to *Nature*. In a 1983 paper, we suggested that the O/M system of the Hadar early hominids represented a unique solution to increased circulatory demands (on the vertebral plexus) that were associated with the origin of bipedalism. We also speculated, contrary to Johanson and White's taxonomic scheme, that rather than giving rise to gracile australopithecines (most of whom lacked enlarged O/M sinuses), *Australopithecus afarensis* may have been directly ancestral to robust australopithecines (all of whom had the O/M system). According to our preliminary blood test, there had been a mix-up at the hospital.

The "Surprising" Black Skull

In *Lucy's Child*, Johanson writes:

> Tim and I had hoped that the Leakeys and their colleagues
> would oblige our theory with some professional response—

perhaps a counterthesis that we could bounce ideas off, even integrate into a more refined synthesis.[12]

The evidence regarding cranial blood flow certainly provided a counterthesis for Johanson and his colleagues to bounce their ideas off of. However, instead of considering that evidence, these investigators ignored it, while claiming to have addressed it![13]

By way of example, according to William Kimbel, enlarged O/M sinuses represented an "adaptively neutral trait" that could not be used to reconstruct phylogenies. Yet, he provided no discussion of the vertebral plexus, or of the connections of the O/M sinus with the vertebral plexus, or of the shifts in hydrostatic pressures associated with changed postures. Having pronounced the O/M sinus as uninformative with respect to early hominid relationships, Kimbel reaffirmed his colleagues' family tree:

> . . . the distribution of venous sinus variants in Plio-Pleistocene hominids gives little or no basis for revising the phylogenetic scheme of Johanson and White (1979). . . .[14]

In other words, Kimbel maintained that robust australopithecines were descended from gracile australopithecines and not (as Conroy and I had suggested) from the Hadar early hominids.

Johanson and his colleagues' failure to give consideration to the physiological, anatomical, and functional evidence regarding cranial blood flow was disappointing, to say the least. In *Lucy's Child*, Johanson states:

> Meanwhile, Dean Falk . . . scrutinized the Hadar skull fragments and announced that the patterns of blood-drainage channels, faintly perceptible on the inside of the fragments, fell neatly into two groups—one looking like *Homo*, the other resembling those of the robust australopithecines.[15]

However, I have never maintained that the Hadar cranial remains fell neatly into two groups. On the contrary, I have emphasized that all five of the scorable Hadar crania (six, if you include Kimbel's scoring of Lucy) have enlarged O/M sinuses like those of robust australopithecines. Rather than being "faintly perceptible," an enlarged O/M sinus is a striking feature and its occurrence in all of the scorable Hadar specimens and all of the scorable robust australopithecines deserves careful thought.

A good theory should be testable. If our blood tests were right, robust australopithecines occurred much earlier in time than the fossil record had yet indicated. In that case, a really old robust australopithecine could still be discovered. And if a robust australopithecine were discovered that turned out to be as old or older than gracile australopithecines, then the Johanson and White taxonomic scheme would be invalidated. In 1986, that's just what happened.[16]

The discovery was a beautiful skull called KNM-WT 17000. It is also known as the Black Skull (because minerals had darkened it during fossilization) and it is just as robust as can be. Found on the west side of Lake Turkana in Kenya, WT 17K (as it became known) is 2.5 million years old, much too old to be located on the robust australopithecine portion of Johanson and White's family tree.[17] WT 17K has a small cranial capacity (410 cm^3) and, best of all, a suite of features that suggest it is descended from at least some of the Hadar early hominids. Bingo!

But there's more to this story. "A robust australopithecine descended directly from the Hadar early hominids, who'd ever have guessed? . . . The paleontological world's on its ear, everything's upside down, why o' why didn't anybody anticipate this find?" complained numerous scientific journalists. The interesting thing is that a handful of workers had questioned the Johanson and White tree and some had anticipated just such a skull as WT 17K.[18] For different reasons, Adrienne Zihlman, Brigitte Senut, Christine Tardieu, Todd Olson, and Russell Tuttle had all questioned the integrity of *Australopithecus afarensis*. (Senut and Tardieu are from the Musée Nationale d'Histoire Naturelle, Paris; Olson is from Albert Einstein College of Medicine.) But because these workers were, for the most part, quiet, methodical, and independent, they did not belong to the paleontological clique that the press usually quotes.

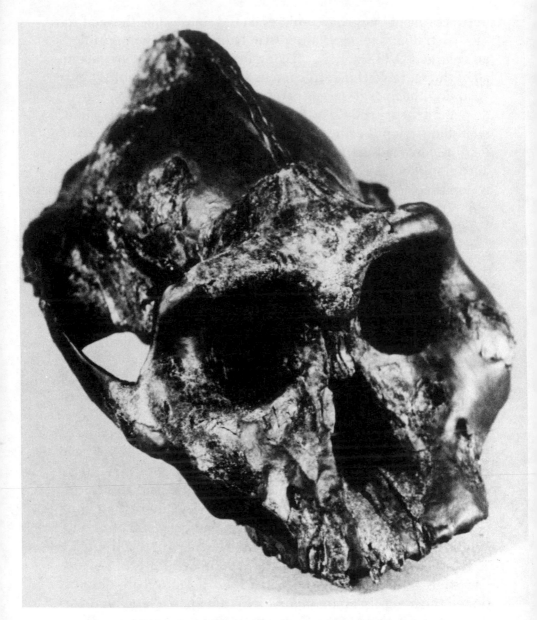

The Black Skull (KNM-WT 17000) from Kenya. This beautiful 2.5-million-year-old robust australopithecine overturned the Johanson and White hominid family tree and demonstrated the dangers of developing elaborate scenarios from insufficient data. (Photograph by Alan Walker, copyright National Museums of Kenya)

This is not to say that the discovery of WT 17K has not had an unsettling effect on the field. It has. Family trees are being redrawn to accommodate the Black Skull, which is generally regarded as intermediary between *Australopithecus afarensis* and the more recent robust australopithecines from East Africa. The problem is what, then, to do with the robust australopithecines from South Africa, as well as the gracile australopithecines. Numerous workers solve this problem by adding branches to their trees—by drawing various species of hominids that evolve in parallel through time. I am skeptical about such bushy hominid trees because they require an awful lot of coincidence. (After all, there's a limit to the notion of happy accident.)

Russell Tuttle is also skeptical about bushy trees:

> Students, teachers, and paleophiles, beware! A new era of taxonomic splitting is upon us. The splitomania, which recently reappeared in Miocene hominid classification, is also infesting the humanoid arena. . . . Several paleoanthropologists . . . now accept no fewer than five species of australopithecines: *Australopithecus afarensis*, *Australopithecus africanus*, *Australopithecus robustus*, *Australopithecus crassidens*, and *Australopithecus boisei*. And we should not be surprised if the recently discovered "black skull" (KNM-WT 17000) and certain other eastern African specimens get dubbed a sixth species (*Australopithecus aethiopicus*) instead of being lumped with an existing species of robust australopithecines. . . .[19]

Functional Morphology Versus Cladistic Analyses

At this point, it may be illuminating to consider the method that most paleontologists use to construct their trees, namely cladistic analysis. Cladists judge the degree of evolutionary closeness of two species by the number of specialized (derived) features that they have in common. The greater the number of shared derived traits, the closer the evolutionary relationship. However, shared traits that are not specialized (primitive traits) cannot be used to assess evolutionary closeness. The fact that gracile and robust australopithecines have five fingers on each hand and backbones are examples of shared primitive traits that cannot be used to assess the evolutionary relationship of these hominids. Lots of mammals have these features. On the other hand, both kinds of australopithecines have feet and shortened pelvic bones that are specialized for bipedalism, and these derived features (plus others) link them together as bipedal hominids who most likely inherited their shared specializations from a common ancestor.

The cladistic method is governed by a very formal set of rules. For instance, one mustn't count each trait that is part of a functional complex separately (i.e., correlated features count once, as a package). Otherwise, one might give too much weight to a single part of the body, such as a tooth that has changed in numerous small ways in conjunction with a particular diet. (Unfortunately, hominid paleontologists frequently violate this rule.) Workers sometimes disagree on whether or not a given trait is derived or primitive which, needless to say, can be problematical for constructing family trees.

However, the biggest problem with the cladistic method has to do with the list of traits that each worker selects for analysis. In order for the analysis to work, one must assume that any given trait list is a balanced representation of all of the independently derived features that characterize the species under consideration. I believe that truly representative (or statistically stratified) trait lists are a rarity in hominid paleontology. One's tree is only as good as one's trait list and, too often (unconsciously or otherwise), workers come up with trait lists that result in the very trees that they have been pushing all along—a sort of designer cladistics. Given these reservations about current applications of the cladistic method, I do not find it surprising that the field of hominid paleontology can be unsettled by the discovery of one new skull.

Although derived and primitive states can be recognized for venous sinuses and other related features, these traits are not proper subjects for cladistic analysis because they are components of *one* functional complex that is involved with draining blood from the head (i.e., the traits are correlated, which is a no-no). However, this does not mean that the features are without evolutionary significance. On the contrary, an effort can be made to understand the evolution of cranial blood flow as a system, and to examine its changes from a functional point of view. This is the approach that Conroy and I have taken. Although our method incorporates recognition of derived and primitive character states, it differs from cladistic analysis in that independently derived features are not enumerated and weighed in an effort to arrive at a most probable phylogeny.

Cladistic analysis is very trendy right now. In a 1986 article about the cladistic method, Randall Skelton and his associates from the University of California at Davis compiled and compared numerous trait lists (and their resulting trees) that had been constructed by numerous paleontologists.[20] They concluded that the most probable tree had *Australopithecus afarensis* giving rise to gracile australopithecines who evolved into robust australopithecines, on the one hand, and *Homo habilis* on the other. The possibility of *Australopithecus afarensis* giving rise directly to robust australopithecines was barely mentioned and then was shown to be unsupported by the brunt of the cladistic studies. Then came the surprising robust Black Skull, looking like a probable offspring of Hadar early hominids—just as the functional morphological approach to cranial blood flow had predicted. Despite this turn of events, the growing vascular evidence is still rejected by some workers.

Australopithecus afarensis: A Species in Question

Because of the Black Skull, few researchers continue to believe that gracile australopithecines evolved into robust australopithecines. Even though the 1979 Johanson and White taxonomic scheme has now been abandoned, some new trees retain a limb with gracile australopithecines leading to South African robust australopithecines and add another totally separate branch with

Australopithecus afarensis evolving into East African robust australopithecines—"splitomania," as Russ Tuttle calls it.

In the introduction to the volume from the 1987 international workshop on robust australopithecines, Clark Howell (of the University of California at Berkeley) states that, with respect to *Australopithecus afarensis*:

> . . . consensus seemed to emerge that this was not only a valid taxon . . . but that a single species was represented by the large Hadar Formation sample, and that the species hypodigm certainly included *both* the Laetoli and Hadar samples (as long maintained by D. C. Johanson and T. D. White, in particular).[21]

I participated in this workshop, and this was not the view I expressed. Nor is it the view of a number of workers who did not participate in the workshop. For example, Senut and Tardieu's studies of elbows and knees suggest to them that both *Homo* and *Australopithecus* are represented in the Hadar material (Lucy falling with the australopithecines). Zihlman also concludes that the amount of variation seen in *Australopithecus afarensis* is too extensive to be accounted for by sex differences alone and that more than one species is therefore represented in this taxon. Sounding the same theme at ground zero, Tuttle says that the Hadar foot bones and the Laetoli footprints are from different critters (with the Laetoli tracks appearing like *Homo*'s).

And the evidence from cranial blood flow? This is problematical when it comes to the question of how many species are really contained in *Australopithecus afarensis*. Kimbel has scored one Laetoli specimen as lacking an enlarged O/M sinus. If he is right, then Laetoli differs from all of the five scorable Hadar fossils (or six, if you count Kimbel's scoring of Lucy). This is consistent with the suggestion that Laetoli and Hadar do not belong in the same species (in which case *Australopithecus afarensis* should be redefined).

The Hadar material itself is another story. All of the scorable crania have robust-like O/M sinuses, and I would call these specimens early robust australopithecines. (Unfortunately, it is difficult to score Lucy for this feature because most of the appropriate part of the skull is missing.) The bottom line on all this is that things don't look good for *Australopithecus afarensis*. Minimally, this "species" seems to contain both robust australopithecines and (at Laetoli) gracile australopithecines and/or *Homo*. Lucy's supposed maternity of *Homo* is therefore in deep jeopardy.

For Lucy to remain the mother of *Homo*, she must have a legitimate heir. And that is just what Johanson and his colleagues claim to have found at Olduvai Gorge in 1986. Reader, I'll spare you the gossip about how Johanson came to work at Olduvai Gorge after Mary Leakey's retirement from that wonderful site. Nor will I dwell on the already too-dwelled-upon conflict between Richard Leakey and Donald Johanson. You can read those details in other books. What I want to address here is not gossip, but rather the evidence that pertains to Lucy's so-called child. To do that, we must first consider the criteria for distinguishing early *Homo* from australopithecines, as well as another spectacular find from East Africa, called the Turkana Boy (or Strapping Youth, WT 15000).

Earliest *Homo*

Any newly named hominid species is bound to be tested by further discoveries. Eventually, the species will either sink or swim. When it comes to the crucial test by evidence, other hominid species have fared much better than *Australopithecus afarensis*. Take, for example, the discovery and naming of *Homo habilis*. The fossil record of this species spans a mere 400,000 years from 2 to 1.6 million years ago. By the end of this period, *Homo habilis* had already given rise to *Homo erectus*. However, the beginnings of *Homo habilis* are murky. Although most workers agree that *Homo habilis* originated from gracile australopithecine stock, exactly when this happened is simply not known. Therefore, the discovered fossil record for *Homo habilis* (found only in Africa) provides just a quick glimpse at the earliest hominids that can be called human.

There wasn't much to go on when *Homo habilis* was named by Louis Leakey and his colleagues in 1964.[22] The name *Homo habilis* ("handy man") was chosen because Leakey thought he had found the true maker of primitive stone Olduwan tools that had been found in the same general neighborhood and credited to robust australopithecines who were discovered five years earlier at Olduvai Gorge. Although a number of skulls from Olduvai Gorge in Tanzania formed the basis for naming *Homo habilis*, they were all distorted or fragmentary. However, cranial capacity averaged about 650 cm^3 in these specimens—considerably bigger than the averages for either gracile or robust australopithecines (approximately 450 cm^3 and 500 cm^3, respectively). Was it not reasonable to think that the brainier new species had produced the associated tools?

Besides having a larger brain, *Homo habilis* also appeared to have larger front teeth (compared with the back teeth) than australopithecines. Nevertheless, the dental characteristics of *Homo habilis* overlapped a good deal with those of gracile australopithecines from South Africa (who, the reader will recall, also had relatively large front teeth compared with robust australopithecines). This led many workers to reject the notion that the Olduvai specimens represented a new species. Instead, they suggested that Leakey's so-called *Homo habilis* was simply a larger-brained, East African version of gracile australopithecine. The future did not look good for *Homo habilis*. Could the new species withstand future tests by evidence?

Those tests came from the Omo region of Ethiopia and Lake Turkana in Kenya. *Homo habilis* held up beautifully. For example, in 1972 the KNM-ER 1470 skull was found on the east side of Lake Turkana. Now known to be just younger than two million years, this specimen had a relatively whopping cranial capacity of about 775 cm^3. In addition to its large brain, the teeth, skull, and face distinguished this hominid from australopithecines. As mentioned earlier, unlike the endocasts of australopithecines, the endocast of ER 1470 also appeared humanlike in its frontal lobe. Further, because of the form of its left frontal lobe, Phillip Tobias and I independently concluded that the group to which ER 1470 belonged may have been capable of some rudimentary form of language.

Today, *Homo habilis* is accepted as the earliest species in the genus *Homo*. Although remains of long bones from Turkana suggest that *Homo habilis* may have been taller and more lightly built than australopithecines, the traits that are most useful for distinguishing earliest *Homo* from australopithecines are found in the skull: Besides having relatively large front teeth, the cranium is larger and thicker and the face and jaw are smaller than those of australopithecines. What identifying *Homo habilis* boils down to, then, are teeth and braincases. Remember that!

WT 15000: *Homo erectus*, Early and Tall

The most complete early hominid skeleton ever found was discovered ten years after Lucy came to light. In the summer of 1984, Richard Leakey and Alan Walker excavated this marvelous specimen from the base of a thorn tree that happened to be using the skull as a flower pot. The hominid was recovered from the west side of Lake Turkana in Kenya and assigned the museum number KNM-WT 15000 (Kenya National Museums, West Turkana 15000).[23] Dated at 1.6 million years, WT 15000 is an almost complete skeleton of a twelve-year-old boy. As is generally accepted, *Homo habilis* gave rise to *Homo erectus*, who evolved into *Homo sapiens*. Because of its teeth and skull shape, WT 15000 appears to be the earliest known *Homo erectus* specimen in this evolutionary sequence (and right on the tail of *Homo habilis*).

Clearly, WT 15000 was an extremely important discovery. It also turned out to be very surprising. By twelve years of age, the *Homo erectus* boy had already grown to be five feet, five inches tall; as an adult, he would probably have reached a height of six feet. Other fragmentary fossils confirm that *Homo erectus* indi-

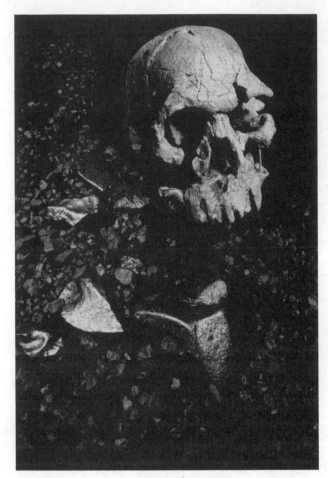

A nearly two-million-year-old Homo habilis *skull (KNM-ER 1470) from Kenya. The sulcal pattern of its left frontal lobe makes the endocast from this skull appear more humanlike than apelike. (Photograph by John Reader, copyright © 1992/Science Photo Library)*

viduals were much taller than anyone had dreamed possible. It is also noteworthy that, unlike earlier hominids such as long-armed Lucy, the arms and legs of WT 15000 were proportioned like those of modern people. Until the discovery of this specimen, paleoanthropologists regarded the tall stature of modern humans as a recent event that resulted partially from environmental causes, such as good nutrition. The lad from Lake Turkana shows us that at least some groups of humans have been tall since the time of earliest *Homo erectus*. So much for the long-held notion that our ancestors were smaller than we are.

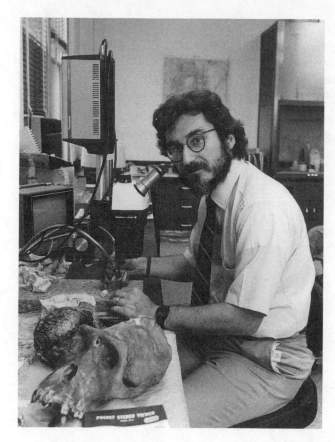

Glenn Conroy of Washington University School of Medicine. Conroy and I took our findings to Nature *(the British journal). According to our preliminary blood test, there had been a mix-up at the hospital.*

brain size ("encephalization") had therefore evolved by the time of OH 62. This reasoning appears to be circular.

Then, there is the thorny problem of WT 15000, the *Homo erectus* boy who lived next door (in Kenya) a mere 200,000 years after OH 62. He would have grown to be six feet tall and his arms were proportioned like yours and mine. And little, long-armed OH 62 (who was approximately three feet, three inches tall) is supposed to have been his ancestor. To me, this seems unlikely.

In sum, the brunt of the evidence suggests that there has been a mix-up at the hospital, i.e., that OH 62 is an australopithecine rather than *Homo*. If so, and if Lucy gave rise to OH 62 as Johanson suggests, then we had best look elsewhere for an unequivocal ancestor for *Homo*. What will it take to convince me otherwise? A skeleton similar to OH 62, but with a relatively complete skull that clearly appears to be *Homo habilis*. Meanwhile, what is interesting about OH 62 is its long arms. They suggest to me that australopithecines slept in tree nests right to the end. Brainier *Homo* found other places to camp out. Places that were on the ground.

And in the sun.

selection for bipedalism in early hominids, as we claimed, why don't bipeds like ourselves have them in high frequencies? This was an important question that required an answer. It was back to the drawing board, and, eventually, back to Africa.

Conroy and I had already learned that when humans stand up, the blood leaving their skulls shifts away from the jugular veins and into the vertebral plexus of veins that surrounds their spinal cords. In fact, this information provided a major clue for understanding the function of enlarged O/M sinuses in early hominids. The question now became: How do living people deliver blood to their vertebral plexes of veins when they are upright, since their O/M sinuses are usually so small? The drawing board where I would first grapple with this question consisted of the gross anatomy laboratory (I was teaching human anatomy to medical students at the time) and, of course, the good old library.

The cadavers and the books both proved to be informative. Yes, the small O/M sinuses of humans are usually capable of delivering blood to the vertebral plexus. However, humans have a whole network of numerous other little pathways that also connect with the vertebral plexus of veins. In other words, robust australopithecines and the Hadar early hominids had *one* enlarged route that could shift blood to the vertebral plexus when they stood up, but modern people have a more diverse, complicated network of small veins that carry out this function. Two different groups of bipedal hominids (one old, one new), two distinct ways to drain blood from the skull. Different systems for cranial blood flow had evolved in different groups.

It sounded good, but could this hypothesis be tested? Because of one saving grace in the hominid fossil record, it could. That saving grace? A few of the many little veins that contribute to cranial blood flow in living people go through holes (foramina) in the skull. These particular veins are called emissary veins and they have names like mastoid (near the back of the ear) and parietal (at the top rear of the skull) emissary veins. Emissary foramina don't exist for most cranial blood veins, of course, but the few that do exist provide a glimpse into the entire system (a kind of window). Best of all, although the tissue which composes veins disintegrates after death, the foramina through which emissary veins travel are often preserved in fossilized skulls.

It seemed to me that one could investigate the evolution of cranial blood flow by determining the percentages of emissary foramina in ape skulls and in the hominid fossil record up to, and including, cranial remains of living people. This procedure has the advantage of combining information from both living and extinct species. I decided to spend the summer of 1984 counting these little holes in skulls in museums in Africa and Europe.

And count holes, I did. Lots of holes in lots of specimens. Whole skulls were examined from fifty chimpanzees, fifty gorillas, and fifty modern humans. In addition, I scored every fossil cranial fragment I could get my hands on for gracile australopithecines, robust australopithecines, *Homo habilis*, *Homo erectus*, archaic *Homo sapiens*, and Neandertals. For good measure, all of the relevant data that could be found in the literature were added to my data and included in my analysis.

Three features turned out to be especially informative: enlarged O/M sinuses and mastoid and parietal foramina.[1] African apes (representing the ancestral condition) had low frequencies for all three traits.[2] Robust australopithecines had low apelike frequencies for the two emissary foramina, but a 100-percent frequency for the O/M sinus.

Results for the lineage leading from gracile australopithecines to *Homo sapiens* were more complicated, however. And more interesting. Frequencies for the O/M sinus were apelike for gracile australopithecines, then fluctuated in subsequently living hominids (never getting above 50 percent), and finally were reduced to very low frequencies in modern populations. The overall trend in frequencies of enlarged O/M sinuses in *Homo* was therefore toward reduction. Meanwhile, the frequencies for mastoid and parietal emissary foramina increased dramatically, especially in *Homo*. Interpreting these data as a window into the entire system of cranial blood veins, it appeared that increased frequencies of emissary veins were probably accompanied by increased frequencies of other nontraceable blood vessels. It was a good guess that the whole system of cranial blood vessels had un-

dition (hyperthermia), the men pedaled on a cycle for twenty to thirty minutes, by which time they were sweating profusely and had an oral temperature of 37.6°C ± 0.18°.

In the minutes following cold exposure or exercise, the direction of blood flow was recorded for the parietal and mastoid emissary veins. This was done by placing an instrument called a Doppler probe directly on the scalp at the point where the vein passes through the cranium. (Four of the men were conveniently bald.) The results were startling. In cold subjects, blood flow was slow and flowed out from the cranium, i.e., from the brain to the skin. In overheated subjects, however, blood rapidly drained from the skin *into* the braincase. Further, these findings were identical to those determined earlier for a third emissary vein, the ophthalmic vein of the face. Thus, when subjects became overheated, blood flow reversed from the normal direction in all three of these emissary veins. Consequently, blood that had been cooled by evaporation from the sweating face and scalp was delivered into the braincase.

Whereas I had merely speculated that the mastoid and parietal emissary veins provided windows into a wider, more complicated network of cranial veins, Cabanac and Brinnel had actually demonstrated this to be the case. They noted that innumerable, microscopic emissary veins exist in humans and that the network of veins found within the bones of the skull itself (diploic veins) opens both externally and internally. By gently massaging the outside surface of the skullcap from a fresh cadaver, Cabanac and Brinnel showed that blood is capable of flowing through this entire network of emissary and diploic veins from the outside to the inside of the cranium.

The three relatively large emissary veins that were used to record direction of blood flow are located at dispersed points throughout the network of cranial veins—at the face (ophthalmic), the back of the ear (mastoid), and the top, back part of the skull (parietal). Cabanac and Brinnel therefore took these three veins to be representative of the wider network and concluded that when blood flows into the braincase in the ophthalmic, mastoid, and parietal veins, it also flows inward in the innumerable other veins that comprise the cranial network. Apparently, cool blood from the entire surface of the human head participates in cooling the brain—but only when a person is overheated. Physiologists call this phenomenon "selective brain cooling." Since Cabanac and Brinnel's original paper, other experimental evidence has accumulated that supports their conclusion (although it still remains controversial).[5] Just like my car, the brain has a radiator!

You can see these cranial radiators at work in any gymnasium. Take where I work out, the Sweat Shop in Albany. Every Sunday, Judy Torel (the owner) teaches a 105-minute endurance aerobics class. The class begins with a moderately paced warm-up. Everybody stays cool. Most people are not even wearing headbands. The warm-up is followed by one hour of nonstop, high-impact aerobics (done to music, something like fast dancing). A ways into it, small sweat spots start to appear on torsos (whole-body cooling has kicked in). Further into the hour, sweat marks are bigger. Headbands go on. At about the forty-five-minute mark, even Judy (who seems not to sweat) puts on a headband. Near the end of the high-impact portion of the class, cranial radiators are in full throttle causing faces to flush as surface vessels dilate and assimilate the cooling effects of evaporation. Some heads are actually dripping. In vessels of a dozen bouncing crania, cooled surface blood flows inward to soothe exhilarated brains. These people are now ready to do weights!

Cabanac's letter had a profound influence on me. In a key portion, he wrote:

> It is possible that emissary veins were developed for the defense of brain temperature. Brain size has increased with bipedalism. The brain's thermolytic (cooling) needs have increased with its increasing size. . . . This hypothesis does not contradict yours but might complement it. I would be interested in hearing from you.

Cabanac enclosed reprints of his scientific articles with his letter. I read them right away and should have seen their implications immediately, but it took three days for the light bulb to go on.

The impact of Cabanac's research hit me in the middle of the night, when I awoke thinking something to the extent of: "Ye gods! Cabanac's work might be the key for understanding why bipedalism preceded the increase in brain size." There was only one thing to do. I got up, got dressed, and went to my lab to plot hominid cranial capacities against the data for emissary veins. It turned out to be worth the trip.

It was beautiful. For the past two million years, the increase in frequencies of emissary foramina kept *exact* pace with the sharp increase in brain size in *Homo*. Clearly, the brain and the veins had evolved rapidly and together. I saw that Cabanac's letter was right and that I had unwittingly charted the evolution of a radiator for the brain in my earlier work on emissary foramina. As Anwander had said about my car, the engine can only be as big as the radiator can cool. Apparently, the same is true for heat-sensitive brains.

But the engine, or brain, and the radiator increased in only one lineage of hominids—that leading to *Homo*. Why? And what about bipedalism and gravity? If the above reasoning is correct, heat stress (or thermoregulation) would have been a key factor in the evolution, and possibly the origin, of *Homo*. As it turns out, there is plenty of speculation, and even some evidence, that suggests just that.

Hot Times on the Savanna

The protohominids who gave rise to the CA around five million years ago were presumably already semierect or preadapted for bipedalism because of their primate ancestry. Like living pygmy chimpanzees, they would have been capable of spurts of bipedalism on the ground or even in the trees. But the shift to full bipedal locomotion would take some time. And during this process, vascular systems would be reshaped through natural selection because of the changed hydrostatic pressures associated with erect posture. Whatever else was demanded of the cranial veins, they had to be able, by hook or by crook, to sustain delivery of blood to the vertebral plexus of veins. Further, because of gravity, this would be true forever after, for all hominids, in all types of environments.

Apparently, robust australopithecines kept cool throughout their evolution. The early ones from Hadar had curved finger and toe bones which were handy for hanging in the shady trees that grew in Hadar's evergreen bushland habitat. According to Elisabeth Vrba of Yale University, the more recent robust australopithecines from East Africa also lived in wooded areas near water. (Unfortunately, the environments occupied by South African robust australopithecines are, for various reasons, difficult to assess.) Further, all robust australopithecines were strict vegetarians, just as Robinson suggested years ago. No need for them to chase down animals during the heat of the day! They had it made in the shade. Except, of course, for the fact that their brains never got very big, and they eventually became extinct.

It's another story for gracile australopithecines, however. Both their teeth and their cranial vascular systems show that these creatures were completely different from robust australopithecines. For example, of six scorable gracile australopithecines, only Taung had an O/M sinus system like that found in robust australopithecines. (And remember, Taung might actually have been an immature robust australopithecine.) Further, the data for emissary veins indicate that unlike robust australopithecines, gracile australopithecines had the floor plan for a radiator network of veins. These are excellent reasons for believing that by the time we pick up their fossil records, robust and gracile australopithecines had been separated for a relatively long time— long enough to evolve distinctly different systems for cranial blood flow.

But how did the division between robust and gracile australopithecines occur? These so-called speciation events generally happen when one subgroup of a population settles down somewhere else. If the new environment (which doesn't have to be far away) is different enough from the original environment and if the pioneers remain isolated from the original group, then the two groups will go their own evolutionary directions. Given enough time, the two populations will become more and more different, until, eventually, they would no longer be able to interbreed with each other (if, that is, they were so inclined, which they probably wouldn't be anyway). At that point, speciation has occurred.

Now, I can think of no better way for a hominid to go somewhere else than to walk there. In fact, by its very nature, any new form of locomotion (be it bipedalism or airplanes) should open up new territory (niches) for more-adventurous souls. Further, we know that a variety of patchy environments were available to hominids during the Plio-Pleistocene. It again appears that Robinson had it right: While robust australopithecines kept cool among the trees, gracile australopithecines ventured afield on foot. Like savanna baboons, graciles spent most of their waking hours away from the forests and woodlands, and on the hot African savanna. It was *there* that full-fledged bipedalism was refined.

And it was on the savanna that hominids experienced the double whammy of changed gravitational pressures on their vascular systems and heat stress on their whole bodies. Presumably, both sexes spent a good deal of time exploiting the scattered resources of open African grasslands that were subject to hot temperatures and intense solar radiation during the day. Many workers, including Zihlman and Cohn, have argued convincingly that sweat glands, reduced body hair, and dark skin evolved as a functional complex in response to the thermal stress associated with living on the African savanna.[6]

Pete Wheeler, as was discussed earlier, takes the topic of savanna-adapted hominid responses to thermal stress a step further. According to Wheeler, early hominids foraging in patchy habitats reduced their heat loads by postural means, i.e., by engaging in increased amounts of bipedal locomotion, especially during the heat of the day, which reduced the amount of body surface exposed to direct hits of solar radiation. In other words, Wheeler sees bipedalism itself as an adaptive response to heat stress. His theory also incorporates ideas about the evolution of sweat glands, hair loss, and even body fat.

Whenever I read Wheeler's papers, I have a flashback to an experience that I had on the island of La Parguera, off the southwest coast of Puerto Rico. During the early 1980s, the island, which is uninhabited by people, provided a refuge for a large group of beautiful, strawberry blond Old World patas monkeys. In their native African habitats, patas monkeys are quadrupedal animals that live in open savanna grasslands. Although well known for being silent, extremely swift runners, patas monkeys frequently assume bipedal stances in the wild. Primatologists have traditionally attributed this proclivity for uprightness to sentinel behavior, i.e., standing up to look out (over the high grass) for predators.

When I visited La Parguera, it was extremely hot. So much so that I could barely function. During the middle of the day, I positioned myself (and a good water supply) on a shaded observation deck that overlooked a large corral containing dozens of patas monkeys. The corral was encircled by high corrugated metal sheeting and, unfortunately, there were no trees within it to shade the monkeys. Although I had read about sentinel behavior in patas monkeys, I was amazed at the amount of bipedalism I saw that day. At the time, I guessed that the monkeys might be trying to see over the tops of the metal enclosure, although it did seem odd because the sides were much too high to allow that. Years later, after reading Wheeler's work, I now suspect that the monkeys were standing up simply because they were more comfortable absorbing less sunshine. (Incidentally, I also think it was inhumane to place the monkeys in such a horrid situation.)

The Radiator Theory in a Nutshell

Put all this information together and you have the radiator theory of hominid brain evolution. This theory explains why bipedalism preceded the increase in brain size in *Homo* and why brain size never got very big in australopithecines. Beginning with the latter, brain size never got above 600 cm^3 because an organism's ability to cool its cranial blood places a limiting factor, or constraint, on its brain size. Australopithecines simply did not have vascular systems that were able to regulate temperature in brains that were any larger. Although robust australopithecines evolved a dramatic, enlarged O/M sinus that delivered blood from the cranium when they were bipedal, this system did not provide a cooling net of veins that could function as a radiator for an enlarging brain. Thus, brain size remained relatively conservative in this group of hominids.

Bipedalism in early gracile australopithecines preceded the takeoff in brain size in their descendants, *Homo*, for two reasons. First, because of the constraints of gravity, bipedalism necessitated a rearrangement in cranial blood vessels. (Since this was also true for robust australopithecines, it was a necessary but not sufficient condition for the subsequent evolution in brain size.) Second, bipedalism allowed the ancestors of gracile australopithecines to "go over there" to thermally stressful savanna habitats. And if Wheeler is right, thermally stressful habitats themselves may have contributed to an increase in the frequency of bipedal behavior. (This is a cyclical, yet logical, notion.) Thus, the vascular systems of gracile australopithecines became modified in response to both gravitational and temperature pressures that were associated with refinement of bipedalism on the savanna. One result was the beginnings of a cranial radiator system of veins in gracile australopithecines. It could do two things: help deliver blood to the vertebral plexus of veins and help cool the brain under conditions of intense exercise. More important, once in place, this system was modifiable. It, therefore, released thermal constraints that had previously kept brain size in check. The engine (brain) could and did get bigger in *Homo*, but only after *Homo*'s australopithecine ancestors had refined bipedalism in a savanna environment that facilitated development of a prototype radiator. That is why the feet went first.

A Fair Hearing for the Radiator Theory

As discussed earlier, my work with Conroy on cranial blood flow was all but ignored by hominid paleontologists. Further, because the initial blood flow evidence was so dramatic, I was pretty sure it would have been widely discussed if our research had supported rather than refuted the (then) generally accepted taxonomic scheme of hominid evolution. Having now formulated the radiator theory, I was faced with a problem: Given the politics of paleoanthropology, how would I ever get this new, more complicated theory discussed? And what good is a theory if it's not discussed?

I knew that for the radiator theory to get a fair hearing, it should be put in a forum where it would be criticized by a number of experts who are knowledgeable about the theory's various scientific aspects, not just by paleontologists with old trees (and reputations) to protect. I therefore decided to submit my theory as a "target article" to the journal *Behavioral and Brain Sciences*. If accepted there, it would not only be published, but also subjected to open peer commentary from many experts, including circulatory physiologists, comparative neuroanatomists, psychologists, neurophysiologists, anthropologists, and paleoanthropologists. They would be tough critics, but I would have the opportunity to respond to their commentaries. Further, my response would be published with the target article and open peer commentaries.

My main motivation for going the target-article route was that I knew the radiator theory would benefit from, and be strengthened by, the cross-fertilization process entailed in open peer criticism. I also knew that paleoanthropologists would no longer be able to ignore the blood-flow evidence if the radiator theory survived intense scrutiny from a variety of scientists, including vascular physiologists.

The radiator theory did survive open peer review. Most of the reviewers were critical but constructive. Many brought new ideas and information to the discussion. Some even suggested interesting new research projects related to the theory. Thanks to *Behavioral and Brain Sciences*, the radiator theory is out and generating discussion, as a new theory should.

Not all of the commentators were helpful in their assessments, however. Consider the comment of William Kimbel: "Falk plunges into pure speculation, propping up a shallow hypothesis with a cartoon-like adaptationist narrative." And Ralph Holloway says:

> At this level of speculation, I could easily assert that as the Pliocene progressed and aridity increased, the distances between shade trees increased and hominids developed bipedalism so that they could stand in the shade during midday more easily, thus reducing the risk of hyperthermia, inadvertently leaving the hands free to make sombreros.

Although these two comments are not constructive, they illustrate better than I can describe the depth of emotion that pervades paleoanthropology.

My Cactus

As Tuttle has noted, the age of "splitomania" is upon us. In keeping with this, it is now fashionable for paleoanthropologists to envision bushy hominid family trees that have lots of branches. A different picture emerges, however, if one ceases to focus on cladistic analyses of specialized features and, instead, considers the evolution of whole, integrated physiological systems. Using the latter approach, details of the circulatory, locomotor, and nervous systems suggest that the overall pattern of hominid evolution was relatively sleek, rather than bushy. The Old Man cactus *(Opuntia vestita)*, appropriately enough, provides a good model for this trimmer view of hominid evolution.

My use of the cactus model is compatible with the radiator

theory and with Robinson's earlier ideas about hominid evolution. Like Robinson, I believe that the first hominids branched into two major groups, robust and gracile australopithecines, and that graciles eventually gave rise to our own genus, *Homo*. From the reader's perspective of the cactus, it cannot be determined exactly when it was that *Homo* budded off. This is in keeping with the known fossil record, which does not pick up *Homo* until about two million years ago. Furthermore, one can see from the cactus that the coexistence of late-living gracile australopithecines (e.g., ER 1805) with *Homo* (e.g., WT 15000) does not preclude gracile australopithecines from having given rise to *Homo*. In other words, populations can continue to evolve after other populations have budded off from them.

The lower, right-hand stem of the cactus contains robust australopithecines from South and East Africa, as well as the Hadar hominids that I consider to be ancestral to the East African population. As far as can be determined, all of the populations on this stem of the cactus were characterized by 100 percent frequency of enlarged occipital/marginal sinuses. If their rugged arm bones and curved finger and toe bones are any indication, the Hadar hominids enjoyed being in the trees, as well as on the ground. East (if not South) African robust australopithecines also lived in habitats with trees and, presumably, shade. Further, all acknowledged robust australopithecines were strict vegetarians. Thus, evidence related to blood flow, teeth, and habitat suggests that the lower, right-hand stem of the cactus, indeed, represents a distinct group of hominids and that it required shade in which to grow (i.e., no thermal stress for this stem of the cactus).

The South and East African robust australopithecines are illustrated as different races of one species rather than as distinct species. (The technical term for race is subspecies.) The cactus is portrayed this way because (with apologies to Gertrude Stein) a robust australopithecine is a robust australopithecine is a robust australopithecine. However, numerous colleagues in paleoanthropology would disagree with this. In fact, as a result of the 1986 discovery of the robust WT 17000 skull (which surprised so many investigators because it looked like a descendant of the

Hadar fossils), some workers now place South and East African robust australopithecines on entirely different lineages!

I believe, on the other hand, that the physical differences between South and East African robust australopithecines exist because the two forms lived in, and became adapted to, different geographical regions, i.e., that each constitutes a different race of the same species. This should not be a surprising concept, since it is one that is used to explain human variation in the world today: Because all living people belong to the same species, *Homo sapiens*, the physical differences that distinguish different populations are due to subspecific, or racial, variation.

The notion of racial differences in robust australopithecines is supported by deep fossil records that suggest regional continuity between older and younger specimens within South and East Africa. In East Africa, the sequence Hadar, WT 17000, ER 406 appears to approximate a reasonable evolutionary lineage. Similarly, according to Ron Clarke (of the University of Witwatersrand in Johannesburg), the South African specimen Stw 252 shows qualities that make it a good model for the ancestor of the robust australopithecines from Swartkrans, South Africa. Presumably, enough contact and crossbreeding occurred between robust australopithecines living in the different regions across South and East Africa to keep these hominids appearing generally similar to each other (i.e., within the same species).

The earliest fossils illustrated on the bottom, left-hand stem of the cactus are the footprints from Laetoli. Since Laetoli's habitat was characterized by open savanna vegetation, and its climate was more arid than Hadar's, this gracile australopithecine stem of the cactus seems to have gotten more sunlight than the robust stem. Scraps of jaws and teeth were also recovered at Laetoli and, as discussed earlier, Johanson and White placed the Laetoli remains together with those from Hadar, Ethiopia in the species *Australopithecus afarensis*. To review, I have separated Laetoli from Hadar for three reasons: First, certain teeth from Laetoli are significantly larger than their counterparts from Hadar. (However, since Laetoli is perhaps half a million years older than Hadar, this evidence could be interpreted as simply indicating evolutionary reduction in size of dentition within one lineage.) Second, Tuttle has argued that the footprints from Laetoli were made by feet that were more modern than those represented by the fossilized foot bones from Hadar. Specifically, Tuttle claims that the curved foot bones from Hadar (good for hanging in trees) could not have made the humanlike prints from Laetoli. Tuttle's analysis does not wash well with authorities whose evolutionary schemes are being called into question, but I find the anatomical evidence that he marshals convincing. Third, the only skull fragment from Laetoli to be assessed for the enlarged O/M sinus that is found is 100 percent of five (or six if one includes Lucy) specimens from Hadar and 100 percent of seven robust australopithecines from South and East Africa was L.H.-21, and this Laetoli specimen was found to lack the feature in question. For these three reasons, I show the Laetoli footprints tiptoeing up the gracile branch leading to *Homo*! (Tiptoeing "over there" to forage and scavenge for food in thermally stressful new environments.)

Another specimen that is high up on the gracile stem is controversial, namely ER 1805, which represents a fossilized skull from Kenya. Some (but by no means all) workers place this specimen in *Homo habilis* on the basis of teeth or form of the skull. However, the endocast of ER 1805 appears apelike in its frontal lobe. I believe this feature characterizes australopithecines but not *Homo*. Hence, ER 1805 appears to me to be an advanced gracile australopithecine and has been so placed on the cactus.

The gracile australopithecines who were our ancestors probably made their living foraging for food or scavenging for meat in hot, patchy savanna habitats. During the course of their evolution, the physiological mechanisms associated with bipedalism became more and more refined. Hair was lost, skin became dark, and subcutaneous fat and sweat glands developed in order to regulate body temperature in new, thermally demanding habitats. The radiator network of cranial veins began to develop. And it may have been this feature, more than any other, that was responsible for growth of the cactus' terminal stem—the one belonging to *Homo*.

The *Homo* Stem of the Cactus

And what a stem it is, as one species grades into another in the sequence *Homo habilis* → *Homo erectus* → *Homo sapiens*. As I noted earlier, it is not known when *Homo habilis* originated from gracile australopithecine stock. We just see part of the *Homo* stem peeking around the rest of the cactus. Members of this lineage coexisted with robust and (I believe) gracile australopithecines for some time prior to the extinction of australopithecines.

Representatives of *Homo erectus*, such as WT 15000, show up rather abruptly 1.6 million years ago in Africa. Not to worry. Since *Homo habilis* grades into *Homo erectus*, the particular species names given to fossils that bridge these two forms is somewhat arbitrary. That is, as more and more fossils are found that fill the gap between species that previously appeared to be distinct, an increasing number of them will appear transitional and thus be named the older species by some workers and the newer species by others. Some paleontologists circumvent this problem by referring to all of the fossils represented by this part of the cactus as early *Homo*.

The approximately two-million-year-old skull from Kenya, ER 1470, is the best representative of *Homo habilis* known to date. However, it is important to note that other apparently early *Homo* fossils (but whose dates are uncertain) were found far from Africa on the island of Java. Perhaps Louis Leakey should have named early *Homo* "wandering man" instead of "handy man," since it appears that it was early *Homo* (perhaps *Homo erectus*) who first left Africa for parts unknown. And a successful wanderer early *Homo* was, because by the middle of the Ice Age, *Homo erectus* had settled in numerous regions of Europe and Asia as well as Africa.

Besides having the proclivity for travel, early *Homo* differed from australopithecines in other important ways. As was discussed earlier, not only had brain size increased in this genus, but the endocast of ER 1470 reveals a Broca's speech area in the left frontal lobe. Because of this, Tobias and I both believe that early *Homo* already had the rudiments of a spoken language. This conclusion is in keeping with findings by Nick Toth, an archaeologist at the University of Indiana, who carefully studied entire assemblages of stone tools from East African sites that date to about two million years ago. Toth concluded that the producers of the tools were right-handed. Since Broca's area and the part of the brain that controls the right hand are right next to each other, it is not surprising to find the suggestion of language abilities and right-handedness showing up simultaneously in the fossil record. A circle of large stones, dated to over 1.8 million years ago at Olduvai Gorge, hints that early *Homo* may even have been capable of building simple shelters! This creature differed considerably from *Australopithecus* indeed.

The record for *Homo erectus* is a long one, since this species lasted until about 300,000 years ago (at which point the record again becomes confused with various specimens that are transitional between *Homo erectus* and *Homo sapiens*). And, *Homo erectus* evolved dramatically during its one million years plus of tenure. Brain size went from around 800 cm^3 to 1100 cm^3, and the skull became long, low, and thick. A fleshed out *Homo erectus* would probably look odd to us with its receding forehead, big front teeth, extremely thick neck, and huge brow ridges over the eyes (with bushy eyebrows?). Even the earliest representatives of this species were taller than their predecessors (recall the Turkana Boy).

But what was *Homo erectus* doing during all this time? Well, making a variety of stone tools for one thing. These included choppers, hand axes, cleavers, scrapers, spheroids, and projectile points. However, this tool kit did not evolve much over time (unlike *Homo erectus'* physique). As one might expect, tools were used for hunting. In fact, *Homo erectus* was the first big-game hunter, and some of his brethren may even have managed to drive a herd of elephants into a swamp at one site in Spain. Evidently, the first true hunter preferred his meat cooked, since the first signs of the deliberate use of fire are also associated with this species. With the hearth goes the home, and it appears that *Homo erectus* lived in huts as well as caves.

Lest we credit this particular hominid with too much civility, we should note one or two areas in which he lacked refinement. Where there are signs of huts (in France), there are also indications that even adults of the species thought nothing of going to the bathroom inside the home. Apparently, toilet training is a relatively recent concept. Moreover, the remains of certain fossilized skulls indicate that *Homo erectus* had the unsavory habit of eating his neighbors. This latter interpretation is based partly on existing casts and records for the important *Homo erectus* specimens known as Peking Man. (Unfortunately, the original fossils were lost when the United States declared war against Japan in 1941, and an effort was made to move the Chinese specimens from Peking to the U.S. for safekeeping.)

Several hundred thousand years ago, *Homo erectus* was in the process of evolving into *Homo sapiens*. Consequently, the fossil record from that time is confused with transitional specimens that can be classified as either advanced *Homo erectus* or primitive *Homo sapiens*. Racial variation is also a factor in this confusion, since these hominids lived and adapted to different environments in Africa, Europe, and Asia.[7] In general, *Homo sapiens* has a more graceful appearance than earlier species. The brain size is larger, with a cranial capacity that averages between 1350 cm^3 and 1400 cm^3. And the expanded braincase is accompanied by a rounder skull, higher forehead, and more vertical face than seen in *Homo erectus*. In keeping with the graceful skull, teeth and jaws are relatively small; and bones of the arms and legs are less thick than those of earlier hominids. And what, among all this dramatic change, is the hallmark of *Homo sapiens*? Is it the big brain? No. This distinction goes to the chin, of all things, which became prominent in association with a vertical face.

One race of fossil *Homo sapiens* may have been sadly misunderstood. This is the Neandertals, who lived between 125,000 and 36,000 years ago. Contrary to the general rule, the earliest of these hominids were not graceful looking. Instead, they had big faces, large noses, protruding jaws, and thick, curved limb bones. These so-called classic Neandertals lived in Europe during extremely cold glacial times, and their physical features were probably adapted for just such cold environments, as experts such as C. Loring Brace, of the University of Michigan, have painstakingly pointed out. Nevertheless, primarily because of their clunky appearance, some physical anthropologists still will not accord Neandertals status as a direct ancestor of *Homo sapiens.* Today, the extent to which Neandertals contributed genetically to *Homo sapiens* is hotly debated. One view, expressed by Christopher Stringer of the British Museum of Natural History and Rainer Grün of the University of Cambridge, is that the replacement of Neandertals by modern *Homo sapiens* "was not an overnight process." Instead, "the real fate of the Neandertals may well have been gradual displacement to more marginal and less favorable environments. . . ." The authors conclude, "Neandertals probably went out with a whimper, not a bang."[8]

Poor Neandertals. They have traditionally been viewed as brutes. At various times, they have been improperly accused of being stooped over, stupid, and even incapable of walking properly on the bottoms of their feet. Today, there are still some workers who maintain that Neandertals could not produce the full range of speech sounds. Is this fair? Not when one considers the cultural evidence, it isn't. Neandertal stone tools, particularly flake tools, were more varied and sophisticated than those of their predecessors. The earliest known deliberate burials are associated with Neandertals, and these were often accompanied by rituals such as surrounding the deceased with animal horns or covering the grave with flowers. Various sites have yielded suggestions of bear cults or hunting rituals that included the use of red ochre. Like *Homo erectus,* Neandertals sometimes ate their neighbors. In short, even if Neandertals appeared a little less refined than other groups of hominids, they appeared to have a relatively advanced culture. They also had the largest average cranial capacity on record, exceeding even that of modern humans.

About 40,000 years ago the weather warmed and, as if out of

the blue, archeological evidence generally associated with modern humans like ourselves appeared. Nobody is quite sure whence came *Homo sapiens sapiens,* otherwise known as Cro-Magnon, or what the relationship of this subspecies was to the earlier-living Neandertals. What is known, however, is that these humans underwent an incredible cultural revolution—one that was so dramatic that the science writer John Pfeiffer has called it a creative explosion.[9] During this last part of the Old Stone Age, tools were more complicated, better designed, and made from a variety of materials, including stone, bone, teeth, wood, and antler. Hunting was still an important way of life and reindeer had become a highly preferred meat, although fishing had also come into its own. For the first time, artistic expression is well represented in the fossil record. Many materials were engraved with artistic designs, and personal ornaments were valued by these people. It is during this time that the famous cave art appears, as well as little figurines of humans and animals. By 30,000 years ago the female Venuses, which some take to be mother-goddesses—and my favorite art—were prevalent. Finally, apparently having inherited the wanderlust of early *Homo, Homo sapiens* colonized Australia somewhere around 40,000 years ago and crossed the Bering land bridge into North America at some point after that, perhaps as recently as 20,000 years ago.

We are at the tip of the cactus and, although it may seem incredible, for all practical purposes one species of primate has taken over the world. I believe that *Homo sapiens* was able to do this because of the evolution of the brain that occurred during the past two million years. I also think that brain size would not have increased as it did in *Homo* if our australopithecine ancestors had not begun to develop a radiator network of cranial veins that could evolve with and cool an enlarging brain. I call what happened to the internal organization of the brain as it increased in size in *Homo* the "braindance."

during neurological development, and the brain began to evolve toward full-blown speech.

The basic stuff of hominid brain evolution probably had to do with the timing of specific events during neurological development. As a result, subtle shifts occurred in at least two related areas—the distribution of receptor sites for neurochemicals and the connectivity of neurons. The steps were familiar, but the timing of events changed the overall dance. As the brain skyrocketed to three times its expected size, other shifts occurred in its overall floorplan. Extra amounts of cerebral cortex appeared in prefrontal areas (where ambition lives and ideas are held on-line) and posterior association regions (for putting everything together).

But the evolution of the brain of *Homo* didn't just take off of its own accord. The shifts in neurochemicals, anatomy of neurons, and so on, provided only the underlying mechanics (or steps) of the braindance. The real cause of this lively jig rests with the behaviors of early *Homo* that were targeted by natural selection. Therein lies the prime mover of human brain evolution.

And the radiator network of veins: What was its role? Certainly not that of a prime mover. Rather, the radiator was a prime releaser. Think of it this way: You've got a frisky puppy and your neighborhood has a very strict leash law. Every day you and your puppy pass numerous other dogs who are being properly walked by their owners. There are no strays running loose. Your dog is a rambunctious thing who periodically hears or smells something interesting and strains vigorously to take off. However, your trusty leash keeps him in check. One day, the two of you are calmly walking down the street. For some reason, you let go of the leash. At first, Fido does not notice and just keeps going at his normal pace. Suddenly, he perceives something interesting and takes off. What caused him to run away? You dropping the leash? No. That merely released him so he could take off. The real cause was the "something interesting" that Fido perceived. Perhaps it was a rabbit or another dog. You're going to have to look around the neighborhood to find out what really moved Fido. Like the dropping of the leash, the radiator network of veins merely permitted brain size to increase in *Homo*. We're going to have to look at what went on during the past two million years to see why it did.

Since the time of Darwin, there have been many speculations about possible prime movers of human brain evolution. Some of these have been rather fanciful. Among the nominees are warfare, work, language, tool production, throwing, and hunting. As one might surmise from this list, more credit for stimulating brain evolution has traditionally been given activities typically pursued by males than by females. Fortunately, this bias is being corrected now that many of the young investigators whose work influences paleoneurology are female. (Women whose research has direct implications for understanding evolution include, among others, Este Armstrong, Beatrix Gardner, Kathleen Gibson, Melissa Hines, Doreen Kimura, Mary Leakey, Marjorie LeMay, Sue Savage-Rumbaugh, Denise Schmandt-Besserat, Brigitte Senut, Pat Shipman, Holly Smith, Elisabeth Vrba, Betty Zimmerberg, and Adrienne Zihlman. Darwin never had it so good! This is not to say that there are no wonderful men in the field. There are.)

Despite all the speculation about prime movers, there seems to have been resistance to the simple possibility that brain size increased as a result of selection for general intelligence. Although it is true that brain size does not correlate highly with intelligence among living people, this resistance is puzzling for several reasons. First, as Harry Jerison (of the University of California at Los Angeles) has shown, relative brain size increased a bit during the independent evolution of many groups of mammals. Since increased relative brain size among nonhuman primates seems to be related to increased curiosity, intelligence may well have been an important factor during nonhuman primate and (by extension) mammalian evolution.[3]

It is also easy to envision the adaptive advantage of intelligence in its multifaceted sense (which is the best way to go, since intelligence is a notoriously difficult concept to define). Hominids that (a) stayed alive, and (b) bred successfully would have been targets of natural selection. Presumably, many aspects of intelligence would have facilitated such selection. For example, numerous workers have suggested that social intelligence was strongly

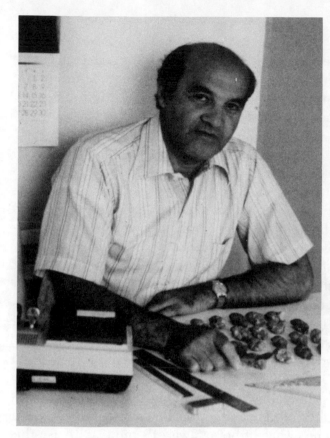

Harry Jerison with an array of endocasts. A leading expert on the brain and intelligence, Jerison's work shows that brain size increased somewhat during the independent evolution of many groups of mammals. (Photograph courtesy H. Jerison)

selected for because socially skilled hominids would have had differential access to food and mates. Similarly, selection for the comprehension and production of speech would also have benefited the early possessors of these gifts. Left-hemisphere time sequencing would have been honed with the refinement of language skills, and such selection may even have facilitated development of the perception of time itself.[4]

With the latter would have come a concept of death (burial of the dead), the ability to worry about the future (e.g., to fantasize escape routes), and a tendency for looking both ways when crossing the ravine (or street). Surely these behaviors were and are adaptive. Humans are speculative, language bearing, and fretful to a degree that exceeds nonhuman primates, including our closest cousin, the chimpanzee. It is time to view these aspects of mind within an evolutionary framework. I suggest that better information processing (or general intelligence) was the prime mover of brain evolution in *Homo*. That's what Mother Nature went for, once the brain *could* get bigger.

Through a Mirror Darkly

Remove part of a person's prefrontal cortex and the person loses ambition, the ability to plan ahead, and, yes, even his or her worries. In this respect, the "me" (or sense of self) lives in the prefrontal cortex. My colleague, Gordon Gallup, has shown that chimpanzees and orangutans recognize themselves in mirrors. Like humans, then, they seem to have a sense of "me." Gallup's recent research (with Jack Maser of the National Institute of Mental Health) suggests that information processing regarding self probably intensified along with increased brain size in *Homo*.[5]

Gallup defines mind (I would probably call it social intelligence) as the ability to (1) "reflect on one's own thoughts and emotions (i.e., to be aware of being aware)" and (2) "to use this capacity as a basis for inferring the experience of others." Although it is a little difficult to investigate the first ability in apes, some ingenious experiments have clearly demonstrated that chimpanzees are capable of the second. In one of the first recorded examples, the late Wolfgang Kohler placed a chimpanzee named Chica in a room with two sticks that could be fitted together to obtain a fruit bait.[6] When it was clear that Chica was not going to solve the problem, Kohler gave the two sticks to Sultan, a chimpanzee who was watching the experiment from outside the cage. Sultan fitted the two sticks together and rather than using them to acquire the fruit himself, pushed the sticks toward Chica. Kohler concluded that Sultan saw "the task to be carried out, from the standpoint of the other animal." Since Kohler's classic work, numerous investigations have confirmed that chimpanzees, like humans, make presumptions about the mental life of others.

However, only humans have evolved social intelligence to the point where they infer the mentality of deities. As Maser and Gallup say:

> ... God, as the ultimate attribution, is a natural extension of our ability to reflect on our own mental states. We typically use these reflections as a model for presuming the mental life of others, but a logical extension of that capacity is to use these reflections to infer the mentality of a theistic entity.[7]

In other words, only humans have the cognitive capacity to conceive of a God, and Maser and Gallup see a sense of self as a necessary but not sufficient condition for this capacity.

Why, then, do humans conceive of a God when, presumably, other animals do not? I think it is because humans have relatively large, time-binding, worrying, planning-ahead prefrontal cortices. As Maser and Gallup point out, once one becomes aware of (a) the self's existence, and (b) death in others, one's own inevitable death becomes a source of concern. Thus, "death is a major motivational component forcing into use our cognitive capacity to conceive of God."[8] Religion (the great comforter) provides an adaptive means by which our species copes with the existential terror that derives from better information processing by our evolved frontal lobes. (Suicide would be an example of a maladaptive way to cope with such terror.)

Maser and Gallup have done nothing less than identify a basic behavioral complex that seems dependent upon higher cognitive abilities that are facilitated by an expanded prefrontal cortex. From a paleoneurological perspective, it is significant that religion appears exclusively and universally in humans. But what of the fossil record? When do the concepts of death and an afterlife first appear? Although a precise answer may never be determined, the fossil record does provide some upper limits for the appearance of religious behaviors.

Certainly big-brained, but beleaguered Neandertals had some sort of religion. As far as we know, they were the first hominids to bury their dead. Times were cold and the earth was frozen hard. Consequently, Neandertals often buried their dead in small graves, with corpses in flexed or semiflexed positions. Despite the practicality of their burials, by 50,000 years ago some Neandertal graves had become quite spectacular. For instance, analysis of pollen deposits from Shanidar Cave in northeastern Iraq indicates that the grave of an adult male may have been covered with an assortment of colorful flowers.

From our Western perspective, we might be tempted to view other examples of Neandertal's treatment of the dead as ghoulish. For example, there's the lad from a shallow grave in Teshik-Tash, Russia, whose remains were surrounded by numerous pairs of goat horns. An equally intriguing find emerged with the discovery of a cave that had been closed for many thousands of years in Monte Circeo, Italy. Within the cave, a Neandertal skull was found resting bottom up in the middle of a circle of rocks. The base of the skull was broken away as if the brains had been deliberately removed.[9] Nor was this the first sign of a possible cannibalistic ceremony in the fossil record! Perhaps as long ago as half a million years, *Homo erectus* had acquired the unsavory habit of breaking into the braincases of his dead brethren.

Although the reader may flinch at the suggestion that cannibalism indicates higher cognitive abilities, historical records indicate that cannibalism practiced by *Homo sapiens* in the late nineteenth and first half of the twentieth centuries served ceremonial more than nutritive purposes. Admittedly, because of their sensationalism, reports of cannibalism are murky and difficult to interpret. Nevertheless, several points of agreement do emerge from the literature regarding the eating of human flesh among Australian aboriginals from a tropical rain forest environment: Cannibalism was a relatively rare event. But when it did occur, women and children were eaten more often than men. And, as one might expect, the victims usually came from other tribes. Furthermore, women or boys seem to have been prohibited from witnessing cannibal feasts. In fact, it is the practice of cannibalism exclusively by adult males that is most suggestive of a ceremonial significance:

... in 1940 ... (when a man was deliberately killed for excessive sexual misconduct), it was necessary that a man drink the blood of a cannibalistic victim before he could attain the status of a *gubi* ("wise man" or "doctor"); it was also reported that anyone who had persistently broken the social code might be killed by senior men of the tribe, the flesh eaten, and the blood offered to younger men to drink.[10]

We, of course, have no way of knowing what *Homo erectus* thought about death or a possible afterlife. We do know, however, that there are a large number of *Homo erectus* skullcaps that look as though they have been deliberately opened. Too many, I think, to be mere coincidence. If *Homo erectus* did practice cannibalism, it could have been for any number of reasons documented in historical times. These include intertribal warfare, personal revenge, punishment, or rituals associated with rites of passage, such as birth, formal entrance into manhood, marriage, or death. Or perhaps *Homo erectus* simply ate the brains of his victims to assimilate their powers. We'll never know for sure. But one thing is certain. Unless the numerous faceless, bottomless skullcaps from Java and China occurred coincidentally by pure, dumb luck, *Homo erectus* did have a concept of death. And that's not bad information processing for 1,000 cm^3 of brains.

Language: "The Rolls-Royce of Brain Adaptations"

But there are earlier signs of better information processing in the fossil record. After all, Toth's knapping experiments with stone tools indicate that by two million years ago, hominids (probably *Homo habilis*) were already right-handed. And one of those hominids, KNM-ER 1470, had a left frontal lobe with the sulcal pattern that indicates Broca's speech area in human brains. Thus, the subtle shifts toward greater brain lateralization had apparently begun by the time ER 1470 arrived on the scene. And you didn't have to have a particularly large cranial capacity to be admitted to

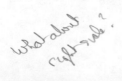
What about right side?

183

the dance hall—ER 1470's was only 775 cm^3. Bigger than any capacity for an australopithecine, to be sure, but considerably smaller than the 1,400 cm^3 average of today.

Harry Jerison calls language the "Rolls-Royce of brain adaptations." I think he is right, for this particular kind of information processing is a luxury item, afforded no species other than our own. Noble machines like the Rolls are not invented overnight. Their splendor is honed over generations, and not without some pride. The fossil record indicates to me, if not to others, that language's manufacture has also been of long and proud duration.

Some of my colleagues would disagree. They think the capacity to make symbols originated in *Homo sapiens* and that this capacity did not emerge as fully reflective language until the appearance of the gorgeous cave art, sculpture, fishing technology, and personal adornment that characterizes the Upper Paleolithic, some 35,000 years ago. Although it is true that the cultural products of earlier *Homo* are dowdy by comparison, a sudden appearance of something as universal and complex as language does not feel right. That is not to say that ER 1470 and his kin had full-blown language. Of course not. But they were in the dance hall and the beginnings of language were there.

The beginnings of language. Now there's the crux. Since primates either have language or they don't, how do we conceive of the beginnings of language? What was the first language, the *Ur-*language, like? And if language began two million years ago, what accounts for its long evolution? Although these questions may seem impossible to answer at first, the dazzling research of one woman offers strong clues for understanding the origins of language.

The Evolution of Writing

Presumably, the first manifestations of language were spoken. This presents something of a problem to those who grapple with language origins. If only there were such a thing as a fossilized remnant of the *Ur*-language or a magic phonograph of speech utterances that occurred in early *Homo*! All is not lost, however, because the evolution of the ability to record speech, or writing, did leave an archeological record. Although full-fledged writing did not appear until about 3,500 years ago, I believe archaeologist Denise Schmandt-Besserat's delineation of the prior stages that led to writing is instructive for understanding the earlier evolution of spoken language.[11]

Schmandt-Besserat, of the University of Texas at Austin, did a remarkable thing. While working in archaeological collections from sites ranging from Turkey and Palestine to Syria and Iran (i.e., throughout the Fertile Crescent), she noticed that little clay objects kept popping up. Nobody had paid much attention to them and, consequently, they were cataloged under different categories in different collections. Thus, one archaeologist's game pieces were another's phallic symbols, amulets, or sling missiles. Schmandt-Besserat found this very curious, so she began a systematic investigation of these little objects. And what a gold mine her research turned out to be! From seemingly insignificant bits of little clay, Schmandt-Besserat's findings have blossomed into a clear exposition of the origins and evolution of writing.[12]

As Schmandt-Besserat has shown, writing derived from earlier record keeping that was invented for very practical reasons. By 5,000 years ago, metallurgy and food production had resulted in the world's first civilizations, such as those developed by the Sumerians of Mesopotamia. Trade was in full flourish, and accurate record keeping had already been invented to keep track of exchanges of livestock and other goods. Obviously, accurate counting was crucial for these records, and counting was one of the earliest precursors of writing.

The earliest known artifacts connected with simple counting are bones upon which sightings of the moon are thought to have been recorded as individual notches. These lunar calendars have been found in caves in the Middle East that were inhabited between 12,000 and 17,000 years ago, and in Abri Blanchard, France, as long ago as 30,000 years. However, concrete counting

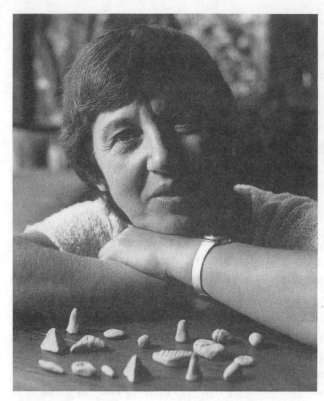

Denise Schmandt-Besserat. From seemingly insignificant bits of little clay, her findings have blossomed into a clear exposition of the origins and evolution of writing. (Photograph courtesy D. Schmandt-Besserat)

whereby one-to-one counting is fused with specific identification of the thing being counted did not appear until about 10,000 years ago. That's where Schmandt-Besserat's bits of clay come in.

Each clay object turned out to be a token. These tokens appeared in a variety of shapes, and each shape stood for a different animal or measure of grain. Thus, three animals could be recorded with three cylinders, three measures of grain with three spheres, and so on. For the next 5,000 years, tokens spread throughout the Middle East, and eventually there appeared new and more complicated tokens to represent merchandise associated with an increasingly complex urban economy.

According to Schmandt-Besserat, Sumerian accountants were responsible for three cognitive leaps that occurred by 5,000 years ago: First, three-dimensional tokens were replaced by two-dimensional pictographs that could be inscribed on tablets with styluses. Second, shapes that had previously denoted measures of grain were impressed on tables as specific numerals (wedge = 1; circle = 10), so that counting was no longer one-to-one. Thus were abstract numbers invented.

Before 5,000 years ago, the only written works were ledgers of accountants with lists of names and quantities of goods. A third cognitive leap led to profound changes in the nature of writing: Two-dimensional pictographs were used phonetically to record the sounds of proper names and then, later, other words. To use Schmandt-Besserat's example, if a syllable in a name sounded like the Sumerian word for "oil," the slashed oval symbol for "oil" might be used in the person's name, even if the idea of oil played no role in the origin of the name. This was the beginning of phonetic writing, which became established by the Phoenicians by 3,500 years ago.

Implications for the Evolution of Speech

Can Schmandt-Besserat's lucid analysis of the evolution of writing tell us anything about whether or not speech had a long evolution prior to the origin of writing? I believe it can. It is instructive that it took up to 7,000 years for abstract clay tokens representing animals to occur after realistic images of a bull and deer first appeared at the entrance of Beldibi Cave in Turkey. It took another 5,000 years for humans to make the cognitive leaps from tokens to two-dimensional pictographs, numerals, and phonemes and another 1,500 years to establish a phonetic alphabet. Even though its domain was visual and, therefore, easily recordable, writing had a long evolution.

Think of how much more difficult the evolution of information technology (to use Schmandt-Besserat's term) would have been in an unrecordable auditory domain than in the visual domain! Human memory would have exerted greater constraints on cultural transmission of new speech technology than on new writing technology that could be remembered in clay. Even though human speech can encode information about shape, quantity, and sound much more rapidly than writing can, the latter has its

187

advantages. As any student will attest, it is best to prepare for examinations by studying written notes and texts rather than by relying on one's memory of lectures—to quote the old saying, "out of sight, out of mind"—and it was no doubt for this reason that writing was eventually invented.

Presumably, there were cognitive leaps associated with the evolution of speech, just as there were for the evolution of writing. Were leaps of speech necessarily invented many times over because of the frailty of human memory? If so, did this slow down the whole process, so that cognitive leaps that occurred during the emergence and evolution of speech were incorporated more slowly into language than were the later leaps associated with writing?

And what about the first words? As the first renderings in clay were realistic rather than abstract, were the first words imitative (or onomatopoeic)? If it took 7,000 years to get from realistic images of cattle to abstract clay-token cows, how much longer would it have taken to get from a realistic sound for cow (perhaps a "moo") to an unseen and unrecorded, yet conventionally accepted, abstract word for cow? It seems that if visible writing had a long evolution, then that of its predecessor, unseen speech, must have been much, much longer. It is therefore reasonable to attribute the increase in cranial capacity that occurred in *Homo* to prolonged selection for better information processing that included a hefty dose of speech. After all, such an honor is only befitting the Rolls-Royce of brain adaptations!

The Art Scene

Between 35,000 and 10,000 years ago, a prehistoric artistic revolution occurred in Europe. During this period, known as the Upper Paleolithic, Cro-Magnon painters, sculptors, and craftsmen created thousands upon thousands of works, ranging from spectacular cave paintings to wonderful little engraved figurines. Some of my colleagues, as has been noted, believe that the sudden appearance of Upper Paleolithic art coincided with the

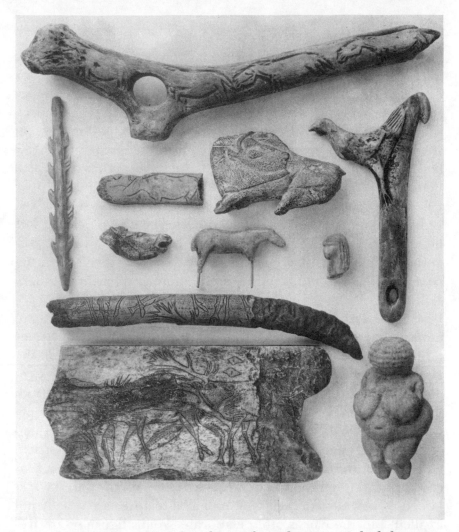

Examples of engravings and sculpture from the Upper Paleolithic in Europe. (Courtesy Department of Library Services, American Museum of Natural History)

emergence of language in *Homo sapiens*. Since I reject this notion in favor of the one outlined above, what does account for the Upper Paleolithic art scene?

First of all, the view that language did not occur until the appearance of art is a materialistic interpretation and typical of our Western culture. (It is also understandable that such a position has its advocates, given that archaeologists, at least, are particu-

189

larly interested in material culture.) There is also an underlying fallacy that paintings and sculpture provide direct evidence for language skills. However, research on brain lateralization shows that this is not the case. Great works of art (including music) pack a satisfying emotional wallop precisely because they largely spring from (and appeal to) right-hemisphere spatial, intuitive, and holistic processes. In fact, artists include more left handers than does the population at large. So, if anything, the Upper Paleolithic artistic explosion reveals more about the state of the right hemisphere than it does about the language-bearing left hemisphere. (However, since the two hemispheres do work together, one could still argue indirectly that right-hemisphere accomplishments would be mirrored by increased left-hemisphere skills.)

The earliest known art consists mostly of vulvas and parts of animals engraved on blocks of limestone, and these two themes —naked women and animals—were emphasized throughout the Upper Paleolithic. I think this tells us a good deal about Cro-Magnon culture. So-called Venus figurines were found from France to Russia. These small, stylized sculptures are simply wonderful.[13] With small heads and tapered lower legs, they stand there naked, demurely looking down. The thighs, hips, stomach, and breasts are enormous, and their arms are often missing or resting meekly on the breasts. Some of the Venuses are knock-kneed, which adds to their charm. Facial features are usually not explicit, but the hair is often elaborate. Venus figurines are frequently associated with domestic sites and are widely interpreted as fertility goddesses. (I sometimes wonder if they might not be somewhat classier versions of modern-day kitchen witches.) One is tempted to assume that Venuses represented the idealized feminine body build in Upper Paleolithic times. The models for these little statues had definitely been well fed, a clear advertisement for the hunting skills of their providers.

This brings us to animals, the second theme. There were plenty for the hunting, including reindeer (a favorite dish), bison, aurochs, ibex, horses, and mammoth. Pictures of animals were engraved on bones, and animal sculptures were carved on weap-

As with contemporary hunting-and-gathering societies, a clear division of labor probably existed in Cro-Magnon times, with men hunting and females and young children gathering plant food. As is also typical of these societies, males may indeed have staged special rituals or ceremonies away from the women and children. There is no doubt that hidden caves would have provided excellent stages for such rituals. Further, since women and animals were the main subjects of Upper Paleolithic art, some workers have suggested that the artists were primarily male. Although one cannot be sure, the suggestion seems plausible because adult males may have been more adept at reaching the hard-to-access inner caves that served as art galleries. In any event, there is no denying that Upper Paleolithic art was breathtaking. However, rather than being some kind of cognitive pinnacle, I believe that it simply represents one aesthetic component of the ongoing braindance.

The Braindance Continues

Not that information processing slowed down during the Upper Paleolithic. Oh, no. By the time the Upper Paleolithic began, *Homo sapiens* had already migrated to Australia and would soon colonize the Americas. With the spread of humans over the globe, speech diversified into regional dialects, and these evolved into distinct languages and, eventually, generations of daughter languages. Meanwhile, back in the Fertile Crescent (as Schmandt-Besserat so eloquently showed), realistic depictions led eventually to abstract tokens and, later, the breakthrough concepts of numbers, a phonetic alphabet, and writing. From there, information processing has sped along.

And it keeps getting better. Now that the telephone, radio, and television have been invented, our species is engaged in other revolutions in information processing. Fifteen years ago, I punched my dissertation data onto computer cards by hand. Today, I can walk into my office, turn on my PC (personal computer) and use a program called KERMIT to hop over to the university's mainframe. Over there, I can crunch numbers to my heart's content or, for fun, check my e-mail (electronic mail) to see what's up with Adrienne Zihlman at Santa Cruz or Bill Calvin in Seattle. Or, perhaps, Stevan Harnad (editor of the journal *Behavioral and Brain Sciences*) will have an e-mail discussion cooking about some aspect of neuroscience that I'll want to join in. (Harnad calls this skywriting.) Once I've collected the gossip and other tidbits from my friends, I'll hop back to my PC and work on correspondence or a paper. Need a graph or some art work? My machine can handle that, too. If you had told me fifteen years ago that computers with these capabilities would be standard equipment for today's academics, I would have accused you of dreaming.

My generation learned to use computers as young adults, which is not a particularly good age for learning second languages. The easiest way to learn a second language, such as French or Spanish, and to end up with a perfect accent while you're at it, is to be exposed to the language at a very young age (certainly before puberty). This thought crosses my mind every time I see one of my more computer-literate colleagues playing at a terminal with a toddler on his or her lap. That kid is going to understand computers, and so will many of the ten-year-olds one sees walking around with Nintendos.

If computers seem cold or artificial, there is another revolution just revving up in information processing at an organic level. This is the human Genome Project, of course. The goal of this project is to determine the exact sequences of thousands upon thousands of genes that reside on the forty-six human chromosomes. It is hoped that this monumental task will be completed during the early 1990s. Once it is completed, the genetic map will dramatically speed the identification of genes involved in human disease. The DNA of medically important genes can then be decoded, and the resulting information used to genetically engineer tools for diagnosis and treatment. (This is already happening for some genes, such as that for cystic fibrosis.) This project is so enormous that it is being divided among different research centers (a hunk of a chromosome here, decode a particular gene there). It is also expensive, with projected costs of $200 million a year. Is it worth it? You bet your life, which could literally be extended by results from the Genome Project.

But there's a darker side to our Western version of the braindance. Vast populations of human beings press relentlessly on the earth's surface, at the very time that genetic engineers are racing to develop technology that will dramatically increase lifespan. Unless population-management policies are soon initiated and successfully employed at a global level, the crunch is going to get much, much worse. Yet a conservative, vocal, and politically active segment of the population of the United States has successfully opposed population-management programs (family planning, choices concerning gestation and the right to die) both domestically and abroad. This is an example of the braindance gone awry. It represents a short-sighted desire to impose particular religious/moral codes on others and, as such, is a frightening distortion of the prefrontal ability to conceive of a God. In the long run, it would be better if our species used its enlarged frontal lobes to plan for the future of an earthly world.

As the reader well knows, better information processing has resulted in other threats to our species. Biomedical engineering has yielded horrible biological weapons, not just medical breakthroughs. *Homo sapiens'* relatively newfound capabilities for harnessing energy and synthesizing materials mercilessly batters the global environment and reduces the biodiversity that is crucial for our continued existence, even as these activities make our lives more convenient (and purveyors of the needed resources wealthier).[15] Finally, despite the recent dismantling of the Soviet Union, there's still the "Big Nuclear One" to worry about. And what a sad ending for the braindance that would be.

The Emotional Brain

Humans must be taught to monitor their behavior in order to get along with others. Thus, a significant aspect of growing up in human society entails learning "to think before you act," or, more technically, to exert cortical control over impulses and emotions. At times, often under the wrong circumstances, the delicate balance between reason and emotion is subject to disruption. And that, as we all know, is when people lose control.

Reason meets emotion in a phylogenetically old part of the brain known as the limbic system. This system is located in a series of structures on the lower and inside surfaces of the cerebral hemispheres, and its primary concerns are emotions, memory, and—to a smaller degree in humans—smell. The limbic system receives and sends fibers to highly integrated association cortices and also has connections with gut-level visceral circuits. One limbic structure, the hippocampus, is particularly important for activating the storage and retrieval of memories. Thus, an important limbic function is to label incoming cognitive (higher) information in light of input from an emotional (gut) level—with varying degrees of positive or negative valence. Another function is to archive some of these sensations in memory, depending on the quality of their emotional labels. The limbic system also sends information about emotional states such as fear or aggression to the cortex, which can then take action.

In the past, many researchers believed that the limbic system was primitive and that human emotions, therefore, remained static during the course of evolution. Este Armstrong, of the Armed Forces Institute of Pathology, however, has shown that the limbic system played an important role during hominid evolution.[16] For one thing, once scaling factors are taken into account, the size of the human limbic system is as large as that of nonhuman primates. As the brain enlarged during hominid evolution, so did its limbic system. Within this system, however, olfactory structures are reduced in humans relative to other primates. On the other hand, there are more neurons than expected in another limbic structure of humans, the anterior thalamic nucleus (which helps bring emotional information into consciousness).

The latter finding by Armstrong and her colleagues is particularly interesting because, for reasons that remain mysterious, a similar trend for more anterior thalamic neurons correlates with single-male (i.e., monogamous and harem) but not multimale (polygynous) mating patterns in nonhuman primates. This discovery led Armstrong to conclude that the integration of learning and memory states with emotions may be set somewhat differently in primates living in different social organizations. Other researchers, working on a variety of primate species, have confirmed the role of the limbic system for maintaining social order. Damage to limbic structures has been shown to alter dominance hierarchies and severely disrupt grooming, sexual, maternal, and other social behaviors.

Whatever its social functions, the limbic system must also have had an important role during the evolution of information processing in *Homo*. According to Armstrong:

> An enlarged limbic system strategically placed to receive a maximal amount of information from the association cortex enables a cultural adaptation by giving symbols access to the limbic system that is equal to that of information derived from sensory systems. This ability in turn permits the individual to focus attention upon arbitrary symbols, to have those symbols satisfy basic desires, and to sustain continuing symbolic/cultural behaviors.[16]

Despite this aspect of the braindance, we must not lose sight of the fact that our evolved limbic systems are delicately veneered on a basic primate brain. Chimpanzees are not very good at controlling their feelings, and inside each one of us there is a chimpanzee screaming to get out. The bottom line is that the issue of cortical control of emotional impulses is likely to be decisive for our species.

even prone toward cannibalism, group violence, and killing each other to settle dominance disputes. Clearly, it is time for the traditional view of human nature to be reassessed.

Dominance Hierarchies:
The Baboon Model

I still vividly recall one lecture that I attended as a graduate student in the early 1970s. It was on baboon behavior, and I left the classroom with a worldview different from the one I held when I entered. Any biological anthropologist of my generation will have heard a version of that same riveting lecture; consequently, its content has left an indelible mark on our discipline.

We learned that certain baboons live in open grasslands (or savannas) that provide environmental conditions believed to be similar to those experienced by our earliest ancestors. Because of an assortment of predators, it is dangerous out there on the African savanna. The saving grace of baboons is their tightly knit social organization. The baboon troop is organized around a hierarchy of adult males who provide protection as the troop wanders in its daily search for food and trees to sleep in. These males are characterized by a very specific pecking order or so-called dominance hierarchy in which each individual knows his exact place with respect to every other adult male. The most dominant monkey in the troop is known as the alpha male; the second most dominant is the beta male. (From then on, primatologists just assign them numbers.)

How do primatologists ascertain the ranks of male baboons? Essentially, they keep track of which animals receive preferential treatment and who takes part in and wins the most disputes. Dominant baboons receive more than their fair share of food, water, and sexually receptive females. They control troop movements and are the first to defend its members in the face of danger. Females, especially those with young, stay close to dominant males.

Subordinate baboons, including females, show submissive

body language toward dominant monkeys. This includes facial gestures (e.g., looking away, smacking the lips, or jerking the head), presenting the hindquarters (which is similar to the gesture made by sexually receptive females who are inviting copulation), and grooming of dominant monkeys' coats. The dominance hierarchy is continually being tested, as individuals monitor their own positions within it and try to displace others in higher positions by picking fights or through other dominance interactions. Thus, hierarchies change over time as animals gain or lose dominance or simply disappear. Anyway, you get the picture. It's a real jungle out there. At least for males.

And what are the females doing? According to the model that I was taught, females do not have dominance hierarchies. Rather, a female's status changes according to her state of sexual receptivity and whether or not she is a mother. Unlike human females, baboon females periodically go into the hormonal state known as estrus and will mate only during this time. Visual and probably olfactory cues clearly identify estrous females who are, well, popular with the males. At the beginning of her estrous cycle, a female mates with less-dominant males, but at the peak of estrus, when she ovulates and can conceive, she is more likely to mate with dominant monkeys, including the alpha male.

Sexually receptive females are accorded higher status (at least by primatologists) than females who aren't as sought after. A female also gets high marks for having a newborn or very young infant. Why? Again, it is a question of being the focus of social attention. Adults of both sexes in the troop are keenly interested in youngsters and seek their company—accompanied by the mother's presence. There you have it. Female baboons depend on their mates and offspring for their status—at least according to the theory that held sway twenty years ago. (But then, think about how a woman's status was measured twenty years ago.) Thus was born the baboon model for speculating about social organization during the earliest part of human evolution.

At the time I first heard about savanna baboons, what crystallized in my thinking was not an understanding of our ancestors' behavior. Rather, what struck me was that the model seemed to adequately explain much of the behavior of another group of higher primates—modern humans! Remember, I was in a classroom at that time and American universities are wonderful places to observe dominance interactions.

Whether one is a graduate student or a faculty member, it's a jungle in academia. At each level of the university (department, college or school, university), decision-making is dominated by a central core of (mostly) males. Students and faculty have designated ranks and the name of the game is to ascend in the hierarchy. Academics, therefore, continually vie for resources and compete with each other for rank. Testing of the dominance hierarchy is actually institutionalized in a tenure system. We have even outbabooned baboons on one point. Our retired alpha males do not lose their dominance. Universities bestow them with an honorary rank—professor emeritus.

By collecting and analyzing biological and behavioral information, much of it within a sociobiological framework, primatologists have recently rectified a good deal of the male bias that was inherent in the classic baboon model, as well as in earlier studies of other primate species. Where once the roles of female primates were written off as passive (or ignored altogether), contemporary workers have used updated field techniques during the past fifteen years to gather evidence that sheds new light on sex roles in various species of primate. So, say good-bye to the unassertive, noncompetitive, and unintelligent female!

Recent studies of apes and Old World monkeys, including baboons, reverse many of the earlier stereotypes about female behavior.[2] Both sexes of some monkeys are motivated to seek status, and females can be quite skillful at manipulating the social environment toward that end. Dominant females bear more healthy offspring than submissive females, i.e., they use their status to gain resources needed to reproduce rather than employing the male strategy of using status to acquire mates. Females may even use sexual assertiveness (read promiscuity) to stimulate more males to help care for the offspring they might have fathered.[3]

Because of female choice (a term straight out of sociobiology), females may also have a broader role than previously believed in determining whose offspring they conceive. Thus, a good friend rather than the alpha male may successfully inseminate an estrous female. Studies of chimpanzees show that females have a more highly developed sense of adventure (wanderlust) than their male conspecifics do, and they might even be more experienced users of tools for activities like nut-cracking or insect-collecting. However, as adventurous and manipulative as female chimpanzees are, it is the males who do most of the hunting. And the killing.

Chimpicide

Jane Goodall's remarkable research at the Gombe National Park in Tanzania has revolutionized our understanding of chimpanzee behavior. These apes, with whom we shared a common ancestor some five million years ago, can no longer be thought of as sweet-natured or peaceful. In fact, Goodall's observations show that they can be every bit as violent as modern, stressed out, technologically inclined people.[4]

Chimpanzees like to hunt and eat meat. They prey on a variety of animals including bushpig, rodents, bushbuck, and, or course, other primates. Favorite primate foods include red colobus monkeys and baboons. Upon occasion, chimpanzees will kill and eat other chimpanzees and even human infants. Although a single chimpanzee may hunt on his or her own, hunting is frequently a group activity that involves mostly (if not exclusively) males.

Chimpanzees are skilled at cooperative hunting. Before starting to hunt monkeys, they often spend time on the ground gazing up into the trees at potential prey. According to Goodall, it seems as if they are assessing suitable victims and their possible escape routes. Just before beginning a hunt, chimpanzees utter grunts or squeaks, and grin and embrace each other. Although they become excited at the prospect of hunting, chimpanzees can be stealthy, quiet, and incredibly persistent as they surround their prey and prevent it from escaping.

Monkey mothers with clinging infants are often the targets of hunts. If a baboon or colobus mother screams, the males of her social group may come to her aid and attack the marauding chimps. This tactic is frequently successful, allowing the mother and infant to get away. At other times, however, there are no nearby males to defend the victims. More often than not, the chimpanzees will snatch the infant from the mother. Several adults males may then tear the victim's body apart and eat it. Although most victims die quickly, Goodall reports that one ten-month-old baboon infant was eaten by only one adult male and was still alive and calling feebly, forty minutes after its capture. (After an infant has been killed, its mother sometimes remains nearby while the prey is being eaten. Consequently, she may herself become a victim.)

Meat is a highly prized food for which chimpanzees intensively compete or beg. Once a kill has been distributed, meat is eaten slowly, as if it is being savored. If the prey is small, a chimpanzee begins by biting open the top of its skull, sucking its blood, and then consuming its brain. In other instances, the skull may be enlarged around the foramen magnum, and fingers then inserted to scoop out the brain, which chimpanzees apparently view as a delicacy.

However, chimpanzees do not just hunt for a good meal. They seem to enjoy hunting for its own sake, as is indicated by the following passage from Goodall:

> On three occasions individuals who were *already in possession of meat* nevertheless hunted again, successfully. Once, as Figan sat feeding on an infant he had snatched from its mother, he intently watched other chimpanzees who were still hunting. Suddenly he handed his entire carcass to Humphrey (who had been begging), joined the hunt, and caught a second monkey—which he then ate. Humphrey once made a kill while still holding a large piece of meat in one hand; and Sherry, holding in his mouth the remains of an infant that he had killed and partially eaten, captured an adult female (its mother) when she ran toward him (avoiding another hunter).[5]

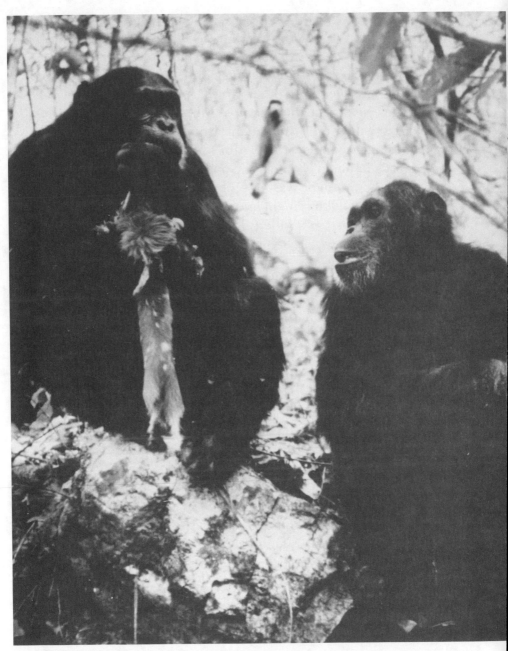

Meat is a highly prized food for which chimpanzees intensively compete. Here, one consumes a bushbuck carcass, while another looks on. (Photograph courtesy of Curt Busse)

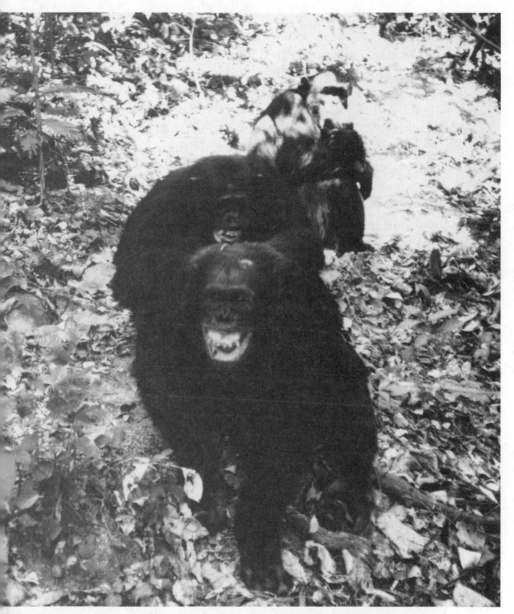

One male chimp grooms another (foreground) immediately after they tried unsuccessfully to gain possession of the carcass from the chimp in the background. Both males are screaming in apparent frustration and excitement over the proximity of meat. (Photograph courtesy Curt Busse)

Surprisingly, the aggression that chimpanzees show during hunting of other species is nothing compared with what they are capable of doing to each other! This is especially true of males, who invest an enormous amount of aggression in settling rank-related affairs. Nevertheless, chimpanzees resolve most of their disputes by threats rather than by actual fighting. However, when fighting does break out over male status, it can be vicious and even lethal—especially if it concerns access to estrous females.

A group of chimpanzees studied intensively by Frans de Waal (of the Wisconsin Regional Primate Research Center), at the Arnhem Zoo in the Netherlands, provides a case in point. In his book, *Peacemaking Among Primates*, De Waal describes the fragile hierarchy between three males, Yeroen, Luit, and Nikkie.[6] At one point, Nikkie was the formal alpha male, but Yeroen was the most successful at mating. In effect, then, they were both the group's leaders. Then Nikkie and Luit formed a sort of coalition that was successful in reducing Yeroen's mating opportunities. Despite this, Nikkie received help from Yeroen that was necessary if he was to remain dominant over Luit. Although he was the alpha male, Nikkie tolerated matings by Luit, and this served to increase the tensions between Yeroen and Nikkie. An uneasy triangle, indeed. Then the hierarchy changed as a result of an unobserved fight that occurred in the night cage of the three males. Luit had become alpha male overnight.

Sadly, Luit's period of dominance, in which "peace and playfulness reigned," was to be a brief one. He died as the result of another unobserved fight that occurred with Nikkie and Yeroen in the night cage. As de Waal describes it, the males' night cage turned red with blood. By the time the staff arrived for work, the chimpanzees had apparently reconciled. Further:

Luit made strong efforts to stay with the other males, which was quite remarkable in view of what they had done to him. . . . Luit had many deep gashes on his head, flanks, back, around the anus, and in the scrotum. His feet in particular were badly injured (from one foot a toe was missing, from the other foot several toes). He also had sustained bites in his hands (several nails were missing). The most gruesome discovery was that he had lost both testicles. All the missing body parts were later found on the cage floor. Closer inspection, on the operating table, of Luit's scrotal sac revealed that, contrary to our expectation, it had *not* been ripped open. Instead, there were a number of relatively small holes. It was unclear how the testicles had come out.[7]

I do not mean to imply that chimpanzees are violent all the time. According to de Waal, when the Arnhem males had a stable hierarchy, violence was minimized. De Waal also stresses that peacemaking behavior is as deeply ingrained in chimpanzees as aggression is. Thus, chimpanzees engage in a variety of reconciliation and appeasement gestures that offset the tendency toward aggression. Under normal circumstances, submissive gestures such as extending a hand, presenting, or whimpering are often sufficient to preclude or end an attack. At other times, making-up behavior between rival chimpanzee males can be more subtle, as the following account by de Waal suggests:

Yeroen, for example, would feign interest in a small object to break the tension and attract his adversary. He would suddenly discover something in the grass and hoot loudly, looking in all directions. A number of chimpanzees, including his adversary, would rush to the spot. Soon the others would lose interest and leave, while the two male rivals would stay. They would make excited sounds as they sniffed and handled the discovery, focusing all their attention on it. While doing so, their heads and shoulders would touch. After a few minutes the two would calm down and start grooming each other. The object, which I was never able to identify, would be forgotten.[8]

If social tensions are high, however, peacemaking mechanisms can fail. The violent interactions between the three Arnhem Zoo males were over relative status and access to sexually receptive females. As Goodall has documented, these are also issues for male chimpanzees that live in the wild. Despite parallels in the political concerns of chimpanzees living in social groups both in zoos and in the wild, it is reasonable to ask whether the violence directed toward Luit might not have been unnaturally ferocious, or even aberrant, because of artificial (zoo) living conditions.

Goodall's work, alas, shows that this does not appear to be the case. Incredible as it may seem, wild chimpanzees are capable of delivering at least as much (if not more) violence to their conspecifics as Luit received from Yeroen and Nikkie. In fact, under one set of circumstances, namely attacks on strangers from neighboring communities, the level of aggression is so high that Goodall regards it as a special form of attack.

Us Versus Them: Male Patrols

Groups of male chimpanzees regularly go on excursions or patrols to monitor the peripheral parts of their range for enemy neighbors. Although they may be accompanied by estrous females who happen to be traveling with them at the time, patrolling is essentially a male activity. Patrolling chimpanzees are cautious and unusually silent, and they avoid stepping on dry leaves or rustling the vegetation. The reaction of chimpanzees upon hearing the enemy depends on how many strangers appear to be nearby. If it sounds as if they are outnumbered, the patrols may retreat silently. However, when the two parties appear to be of similar size, members of both sides display in wild outbursts of vocalizing, throwing, and drumming. Frequently, these challenges end with the two parties withdrawing noisily to their respective core areas.

But woe to the lone chimpanzee who is caught traveling alone or with an infant because, as Goodall puts it, chimpanzees appear to have "an inherent dislike or 'hatred' of strangers." Repeated observations by Goodall's assistants have documented the manner in which patrolling males assault their male and female victims: The attacks were gang attacks of long duration. In all of the incidents, the strangers were held to the ground by some chimpanzees, while others hit, bit, stamped upon, and pounded the victims. The strangers were also dragged about. Although the victims eventually gave up and crouched or lay passively, the attacks continued until the victims were completely immobilized, if not dead. Significantly, the field assistants who observed these attacks believed that the chimpanzees were trying to kill their victims. On several occasions, the aggressors later returned to the scenes of the violence to search for or inspect the bodies of their victims.

In her impressive volume, Goodall meticulously documents a series of aggressive interactions that led to the complete annihilation of one chimpanzee community (the Kahama) by males from another (the Kasakela). What does she make of this? Goodall believes that chimpanzees should be considered territorial, although she notes that they differ in some ways from classically territorial animals. For example, rather than simply chasing trespassers out of their territories, chimpanzees create opportunities for encountering strangers by patrolling peripheral areas about once every four days. Furthermore, adult males behave as if they *like* aggressive encounters. The violence of their hostility toward neighbors and the fact that they will make raids into the core areas of other communities also distinguishes chimpanzees from other territorial animals. In other words, chimpanzees are not just territorial. When it comes to strangers, they seem almost to have a bloodlust. Goodall stops short of attributing warfare to chimpanzees, reasoning that language which is necessary, is absent. I'm not so sure. Although their aggression is not corticalized with verbal strategies or modified weapons, it seems to me that our chimpanzee cousins do a chillingly efficient job of waging war. And I, for one, believe that the Common Ancestor (CA) of chimpanzees and humans is probably responsible for the human taste for warfare.[9]

Homicide

As mentioned earlier, many social anthropologists argue against a biological or evolutionary basis for human violence. Instead, they extol the gentle nature of modern primitives who live in simple nonintensive foraging/horticultural societies (sometimes called bands), and they make the claim that these societies reflect social organization as it prevailed during most of hominid evolution. This level of organization is frequently described as egalitarian, because male status is de-emphasized, and sharing and crosscutting ties with other groups are encouraged. In other words, the norms of cooperation and communal sharing are said to be extremely strong in these simplest societies. Thus, according to Bruce Knauft of Emory University, the !Kung of southern Africa are known as "harmless people," the Semai from Malaya as "nonviolent people," the Waorani of Ecuador as a "tribe where harmony rules," and Eskimo relations are described as "never in anger."[10]

Knauft's own research is on the Gebusi, a small, opportunistic hunting-and-foraging/horticultural society that lives in lowland New Guinea. Knauft describes male social life among the Gebusi as markedly devoid of hierarchical relationships and rivalry. In this peace-loving society, diffuse friendship and camaraderie are the stated norms, and anger is viewed as antisocial and threatening to communal sociality. Yet, despite their apparent gentleness, the homicide rate among the Gebusi is one of the highest ever reported for any society!

According to Knauft, homicide among the Gebusi is primarily a male activity. Almost two-thirds of middle-aged men from two communities have committed homicide, "including some who were among the least assertive and aggressive even by Gebusi standards."[11] Of nearly four hundred deaths surveyed, about one-third were homicides. Although a certain number of deaths (less than 10 percent) occur in bow-and-arrow encounters between Gebusi from different settlements, the most frequent context for homicide is the killing of a man or woman for allegedly being a sorcerer who caused the sickness and death of another person.

Knauft believes that few Gebusi actually practice sorcery. Nevertheless, when someone becomes ill and dies, his or her death is frequently attributed to a male or female sorcerer. Aggressive or assertive individuals are likely targets for such accusations. An accused individual must undergo public divinations and is subject to a swift, violent death if found guilty. As Knauft points out, Gebusi violence thus acts as a strong leveling mechanism that discourages the emergence of assertiveness and reinforces the norms of sociality and sharing.

But what is Gebusi homicide really about? Knauft's careful analysis reveals an answer, of which the Gebusi themselves are apparently unaware: Violence is ultimately about male control of women. For example, the killing of sorcerers is statistically correlated with lack of reciprocity in exchange of sisters for marriage. Significantly, Knauft notes that other gentle societies such as the !Kung, Central Eskimo, and Semai also engage in extreme violence in disputes over female sexuality. Although simple societies may lack the resources (including leadership) for waging much in the way of war, lethal violence is no stranger. As de Waal documented for the chimpanzees at the Arnhem Zoo, tensions over heterosexual access frequently erupt between human males living in simple societies.

Knauft has used his data for the Gebusi to test the controversial sociobiological hypothesis regarding violence. A basic tenet of sociobiology is that animals, including humans, behave in ways that maximize their reproductive fitness, either through producing offspring themselves or by facilitating reproduction in relatives such as siblings or cousins. According to this hypothesis, humans should avoid killing their relatives. Also, if violence is adaptive, one would expect those who commit homicide to leave more offspring than other people. And, indeed, the sociobiological hypothesis was confirmed for at least one group of people when Napoleon Chagnon (currently of the University of California at Santa Barbara) found that killers from a South American tribe (the Yanomamo) have over twice as many wives and three times as many children as nonkillers. However, Knauft's data fail to confirm the sociobiological hypothesis. In fact, contrary to sociobiological expectations, Knauft found a statistically significant correlation between homicide and genealogical relatedness (i.e., Gebusi tend to kill their relatives)!

Knauft's work on the Gebusi is extremely important and has received a good deal of attention. Unfortunately, debate on the sociobiological implications of the Gebusi data has been prevalent in the discussions about his research and this has clouded understanding of its *biological* significance. In fact, Knauft himself emphasizes the interrelationship of cultural, ecological, and sociological constraints on Gebusi violence, but he seems to have thrown biology out with sociobiology.

The extreme violence practiced by the Gebusi and other seemingly gentle societies supports the contention that aggression is a basic component of human nature that emerges in some form, regardless of the explicit cultural constraints on violence. This conclusion is strengthened by the fact that, universally, males apparently kill each other over (among other issues) heterosexual access. Furthermore, that Gebusi men are prone to killing their own sisters as a means of taking vengeance on their brothers-in-law does not negate the general validity of sociobiological explanations of violence.

It matters not a whit, of course, whether there is or is not a human (or chimpanzee) gene for homicide. What does matter is that men the world round are predisposed toward lethal aggression. Furthermore, the assertion that violence is strictly culturally determined is not going to change things.[12] Just as chimpanzee males cheerfully patrol the periphery looking for rumbles, so do human males. And these males even call themselves "civilized."

Murder in Detroit

Nonmilitaristic lethal violence is not just a product of *simple* human societies, as Martin Daly and Margo Wilson (both of

McMaster University) document thoroughly in their fascinating book, *Homicide.*[13] Homicides occur in all cultures. Among industrialized nations, homicides are particularly frequent in the United States, where there are approximately sixty per day. As with the Gebusi, it is enlightening to see who kill whom within civilized societies and why. Daly and Wilson's approach to this question is informed by evolutionary biology and the framework within which they formulate their conclusions is unabashedly sociobiological.

I asked several colleagues to guess what the most prevalent relationship is between murderers and their victims in the United States. Their answers varied. One said "relatives," and another said "strangers, because I think most would have to do with theft or robberies." Another (newly wed) suggested "domestic violence between husbands and wives." In fact, the answer is quite different from any of the above, and very interesting.

In keeping with the sociobiological hypothesis of violence, few Americans kill relatives who share their genes. Of 508 homicides in Detroit surveyed by Daly and Wilson, only 6 percent involved blood kin. Upon further analysis, the Detroit data proved to be typical for American homicides. Thus, "blood relationships are much less lethal than other intimate relationships."[14]

The main cause of lethal violence wherever homicide rates are high, including the United States, is trivial altercations between males. Swift, violent death can result from amazingly minor disputes over such issues as a parking space, access to a pool table, or a macho barroom boast. Although these proximate causes seem incredibly insignificant, Daly and Wilson offer a perceptive analysis that makes sense of these homicides:

> In most social milieus, a man's reputation depends in part upon the maintenance of a credible threat of violence. Conflicts of interest are endemic to society, and one's interests are likely to be violated by competitors unless those competitors are *deterred*. Effective deterrence is a matter of convincing our rivals that any attempt to advance their interests at our expense will lead to such severe penalties that the competitive

gambit will end up a net loss which should never have been undertaken.[15]

Although Daly and Wilson conclude that machismo behavior probably increased reproductive fitness during most of human history, they think its utility has been mitigated in modern societies, where states have assumed a monopoly on the "legitimate" use of violence.

Daly and Wilson conclude their book by noting that homicide rates have fallen in historical times in most state societies. They add that twentieth-century humans may have a better chance of dying peacefully in bed than did their hominid predecessors. But then the authors probably did not know about a United States military plan called "Treetop."

Patrolling the Last Frontier

Just as male chimpanzees love to patrol their borders, so do human males (sometimes with the help of females). The difference is that men, with their fancy neocortices and language, provide rationalizations for why they patrol. Thus, civilized humans patrol in the name of loved ones, or country, or freedom, or God's will, or—my favorite—peace. But patrol they do. When chimpanzees find an unfortunate stranger, the marauding group holds their victim to the ground and attacks him or her with their hands and feet and teeth. They do not stop until the victim is completely incapacitated or dead. Because of their evolved brains, men have been able to replace extremities and teeth with technologically advanced weapons that are both convenient and ruthlessly lethal. And because of their chimpanzeelike natures, they cannot resist these and other military endeavors.

Take, for example, Americans. They have invested heavily in the patrol.[16] In 1982, a secret agency called the Defense Mobilization Planning Systems Agency was created and instructed to report to then–Vice President Bush. By the time Bush assumed the presidency in 1989, more than $3 billion had been spent to upgrade the command, control, and communications technology associated with the United States' strategy for surviving a nuclear attack. That strategy is known in "militarese" as COG, short for "continuity of government." And what a plan it is.

The COG plan for what happens to government officials in the event of a nuclear attack is known as "Treetop." According to this plan, the president will be evacuated from the White House (assuming that's where he is) by helicopter. He will probably fly directly to a National Emergency Airborne Command Post, known as "kneecap." There are four kneecaps, or Boeing 747s, that have been customized with specialized telecommunications equipment. One is kept flying at all times, and another is always waiting at Andrews Air Force Base, less than ten minutes from the White House. With refueling, the "kneecap" could serve as an airborne command post, from which the president would be able to direct military and civilian operations.

The president could also take up residence in the well-provisioned Mount Weather command bunker in Virginia or in one of approximately fifty fallout-resistant command bunkers that have apparently been equipped to act as emergency White Houses. To diminish the chances of sustaining direct hits, these bunkers are secretly located across the United States. One underground bunker whose location is not so secret is Raven Rock, near Camp David, Maryland. During the nuclear holocaust, its lucky inhabitants would be able to enjoy a racquetball court, chapel, laundry, medical clinic, and a barber shop. (Now that's what I call optimism.)

Who are the lucky residents of American fallout-resistant bunkers going to be? First of all, there would be the president and a dominance hierarchy of 17 government officials who are designated (in serial order) as his potential successors. Then, there are 46 key Pentagon officials who would be airlifted to the relative safety of the bunkers, any time, day or night. Another 248 relief specialists and senior Pentagon officials may join them, but only during working hours. In all, the plan is for over 1,000 military and political officials to be evacuated.

If all of this sounds as if the military intends to protect itself in the case of Armageddon, that is far from the stated rational for "Treetop." Former President Reagan, for instance, believed that a nuclear war would be winnable, but only if government leaders survived. Furthermore, there is the added notion that government leaders must survive in order to halt the aggression and to help civilians.

But these noble motives weaken somewhat when one examines the highly sensitive issue of what the United States chooses to target with its own nuclear weapons. As of 1989, the United States was reported to be drastically changing its strategy for fighting a nuclear war with the Soviet Union.[17] The new plan, called the Strategic Integrated Operations Plan (or SIOP-7), calls for development of devastating weapons that can penetrate the deepest military bunkers, thereby removing Soviet leadership shortly after the onset of conflict. In order to facilitate this goal, the United States would plant remote sensing devices inside Soviet territory. Critics of SIOP-7 point out that such tactics might "upset the fragile balance of terror," and increase the chances of an inadvertent launch of nuclear missiles by nervous Soviet Union leaders operating under siege constraints. They also note that the elimination of the USSR's leadership would leave no one to halt the Soviet side of the conflict.

The recent dramatic upheaval in the Soviet Union has created a new quandary for U.S. military experts. As this book goes to press, officials are uncertain about who controls the Soviet arsenal of 28,000 nuclear weapons. The Bush Administration has expressed its hopes that these weapons will remain under a central command authority rather than under the control of numerous independent Soviet republics.

In February 1990, Senator Sam Nunn (a Democrat from Georgia) called for a fail-safe review of the mechanisms for ensuring nuclear safeguards.[18] It was Nunn's hope that the Pentagon would reverse its long-standing objections to new technology that would allow United States missiles to be called back (or destroyed) after they had been launched. He also suggested that it would be prudent to share such fail-safe technology with the Soviet Union. The most amazing revelation associated with Nunn's proposal is that senior American military officials have apparently been resistant to calls for further nuclear safeguards.

These facts represent bits and pieces about (usually) secret American military operations that have been gleaned by the media. Despite the paucity of public information, the overwhelming impression one receives, reinforced by the recent war with Iraq, is that military leaders take pride in and enjoy what they do. Indeed, the recent rapprochement between the United States and the Soviet Union (not to mention the reunification of Germany) threatens long-standing positions of military interests worldwide. Whether disarmament is the next step is another, deeper question that goes to the heart of our views of our species and our apparent predilection for aggressive behavior.[19]

Although the cerebral cortex may be evolved in humans, the limbic system still divides the universe into us and them. Men *will* patrol their borders. And more. Like Goodall's chimpanzees, human beings are neither reluctant to penetrate the territories of others or to use lethal force against strangers. The contributions of the human neocortex are in the areas of weaponry, verbal strategy, and the fact that men frequently do violence to others in the name of God.

One may choose to believe that the parallels between aggressive behavior in ourselves and chimpanzees are just coincidence. It does not matter. Whatever the mix between biological and cultural factors, human beings are aggressive, territorial primates who, resources permitting, venerate their dominance hierarchies within, and seek the thrill of patrolling the periphery without. Although males usually engage in these activities, it is entire societies that support them. In simplest terms, human behavior suggests that, without a "them" to worry about, the "us" would be most unfulfilled.[20]

The Last Dance?

Two million years of natural selection for better information processing has given our species a marvelous brain. Because of its size and wiring and delicate balance of neurochemicals, humans pursue wonderful activities—like worrying about whether or not the cosmos has an origin or trying to find a still larger prime number. People weep at sad movies, write poetry, and laugh uproariously at funny jokes. They listen to music, paint murals, and are capable of seeing the solution to a problem in an intuitive flash. They also make the best damned tap dancers. And all because of the braindance.

But our lovely cortices are veneered over a brain that is constructed according to a basic primate floorplan. The limbic system looms, ever in the background, and our males (and sometimes females) cannot keep themselves from patrolling the borders. Society has encouraged them, of course, by supporting development of what may soon become a global nuclear "Fright Machine" that is not fail-safe against the wrong leader hearing doomsday instructions from the Almighty, at the wrong time. Although the cortical mechanisms for controlling aggression are part of the neurological package that we inherited from our hominid ancestors, our species must vigilantly exercise those controls over our natural primate tendencies to engage in potentially catastrophic dominance interactions. We, therefore, must question which one will ultimately win out—the braindance, or the brainwar.

In her chapter on territoriality, Jane Goodall says of the chimpanzee:

> If ever he develops the power of language—and, as we have seen, he stands close to that threshold, too—might he not push open the door and wage war with the best of us?[21]

In my opinion, he has developed language and (to quote the immortal Pogo) "he is us." All things considered, since *Homo sapiens* appears to have a strong predilection for potentially catastrophic aggression, perhaps the best we can hope for is that our species continues to exert control over its limbic impulses.

Then, at least, we stand a chance of being jolly enemies *forever more more more.*

Notes and References

1: Foraging in the Red Cave

1. R. Dart, *Adventures with the Missing Link* (New York: Random House, 1959).

2. ibid., 10.

3. R. A. Dart, "*Australopithecus africanus:* The man-ape of South Africa," *Nature* 115 (1925):195–99.

4. J. T. Robinson, "Adaptive radiation in the australopithecines and the origin of man," in F. C. Howell and F. Bourlieve, eds., *African Ecology and Human Evolution* (Chicago: Aldine, 1963), 385–416.

5. G. Findlay, *Dr. Robert Broom, F. R. S.: Palaeontologist and Physician/1866–1951* (Cape Town: A. A. Balkema, 1972).

6. Recently, this idea has been eloquently elaborated by R. A. Foley and P. C. Lee in "Finite social space, evolutionary pathways, and reconstructing hominid behavior," *Science* 243 (1989):901–6.

7. This suggestion was presented by several workers who attended the International Workshop on the Evolutionary History of the Robust Australopithecines, at the State University of New York, Stony Brook, from March 27 through April 2, 1987. See also F. Grine, ed., *The Evolutionary History of "Robust" Australopithecines* (New York: Aldine de Gruyter, 1989).

8. R. L. Susman, "Hand of *Paranthropus robustus* from Member I, Swartkrans: Fossil evidence for tool behavior," *Science* 233 (1989):781–84. Susman recently analyzed several finger bones from a South African site named Swartkrans, dated to 1.8 million years ago. He believes the bones are those of robust australopithecines and that they indicate the hand of this early hominid was capable of making tools, "possibly for plant procurement and processing." In keeping with this, Susman concludes that lack of tool behavior was not responsible for the extinction of robust australopithecines and, further, that the acquisition of tools was not responsible for the emergence of *Homo*. Even more tantalizing is the somewhat oblique suggestion that robust australopithecines may have used fire for cooking, protection against predators, or warmth, in C. K. Brain and A. Sillen, "Evidence from the Swartkrans cave for the earliest use of fire," *Nature* 336 (1988):464–66. The problem with this interpretation is that *Homo* was at Swartkrans too and it is not known if one or both hominids used fire.

9. In hindsight, this observation was a little harsh. I've since learned that some curators, such as Bob Brain of the Transvaal Museum, are fastidious about never excluding qualified workers from their collections. In fact, I would never have been able to carry out my research without the access to fossil hominids that was kindly extended to me by Brain, Phillip Tobias, and Richard Leakey.

10. In a letter dated January 16, 1991, Bob Brain informed me that the Red Cave is no more! Most of the research departments of the Transvaal Museum have now moved to a new building behind the museum. According to Brain, the hominid fossils "are now housed in another strongroom which is still a bit sterile but which, it is hoped, will acquire some atmosphere before long. Our new Curator of Palaeontology is Dr. Francis Thackeray and he will be attending to the aesthetics of a new hominid cavern."

11. During hominid evolution, the lunate sulcus was pushed toward the back by expansion of the parietal association cortex, which is concerned with higher integrative functions.

12. The line of reasoning used by Holloway here is a logical error that is called resorting to higher authority or the *argumentum ad verecundiam.*

13. R. L. Holloway, "Revisiting the South African Taung australopithecine endocast: The position of the lunate sulcus as determined by the stereoplotting technique," *American Journal of Physical Anthropology* 56 (1981):43–58; see p. 50.

14. R. L. Holloway, "The role of human social behavior in the evolution of the brain," Forty-third James Arthur Lecture (New York: The American Museum of Natural History, 1975), 11–12.

15. R. L. Holloway, "Revisiting the South African Taung australopithecine endocast: The position of the lunate sulcus as determined by the stereoplotting technique." *American Journal of Physical Anthropology* 56 (1981):43–58; see p. 49.

16. D. Falk, "Apples, oranges, and the lunate sulcus," *American Journal of Physical Anthropology* 67 (1985):313–15; see p. 315.

17. D. Falk, "Hadar AL 162-28 endocast as evidence that brain enlargement preceded cortical reorganization in hominid evolution," *Nature* 313 (1985):45–47.

18. R. L. Holloway, "Cerebral brain endocast pattern of *Australopithecus afarensis* hominid," *Nature* 303 (1983):420–22.

2: Taung Goes to St. Louis

1. Thank you, NIH (RO1 NS 24904).

2. H. Jerison's book, *Evolution of the Brain and Intelligence* (New York: Academic Press, 1973) is a classic. For a discussion of allometric scaling of the brain, see H. Jerison, "Allometry, brain size, cortical surface, and convolutedness," in E. Armstrong and D. Falk, eds., *Primate Brain Evolution: Methods and Concepts* (New York: Plenum Press, 1982), 77–84.

3. For details see D. Falk, C. Hildebolt, and M. W. Vannier, "Reassessment of the Taung early hominid from a neurological perspective," *Journal of Human Evolution* 18 (1989):485–92.

4. K. Zilles, E. Armstrong, A. Schleicher, and H. Kretschmann, "The human pattern of gyrification in the cerebral cortex," *Anatomy and Embryology* 179 (1988):173–79.

5. See E. Armstrong, K. Zilles, M. Curtis and A. Schleicher, "Cortical folding, the lunate sulcus, and the evolution of the human brain," *Journal of Human Evolution* 20 (1991):341–48; H. J. Jerison, "Fossil evidence on the evolution of the neocortex," in E. G. Jones and A. Peters, eds., *Cerebral Cortex*, vol. 8A (New York: Plenum Press, 1990), 285–309.

6. The oldest known *Homo habilis* specimens are dated to approximately two million years BP (before present). *Homo erectus* was already on the scene by 1.6 million years ago.

3: Chimp Brain, Human Brain

1. The information presented here is from E. S. Savage-Rumbaugh and D. Rumbaugh, "The invention of language." Paper presented at the Wenner-Gren International Symposium on Tools, Language and Intelligence: Evolutionary Implications, Cascais, Portugal (1990). Sue Savage-Rumbaugh's comments at the symposium are also included.

2. Drs. Gibson and Boesch were both participants in the Wenner-Gren symposium noted above.

3. The illustration was modified after W. Penfield and T. Rasmussen, *The Cerebral Cortex of Man* (New York: Hafner Publishing Company, 1968.)

4. The homunculus is based on my modification of Penfield's classic maps. It is greatly simplified and over generalized. In order to maintain continuity, some artistic license has been taken. For example, the tongue is shown protruding from the mouth, rather than as a separate structure located beneath the face representation. In reality, there are multiple representations for certain parts of the body, such as the hand, and sensory and motor areas overlap and

differ more from each other than is apparent from this illustration. The relative sizes of body parts also differ from person to person.

5. For details, see K. Zilles, E. Armstrong, A. Schleicher, and H. J. Kretschmann, "The human pattern of gyrification in the cerebral cortex," *Anatomy and Embryology* 179 (1988):173–79.

6. P. S. Goldman-Rakic, "Circuitry of primate prefrontal cortex and regulation of behavior by representational memory," in V. B. Mountcastle, F. Plum, and S. R. Geiger, *Handbook of Physiology— The Nervous System V* (Bethesda, MD: American Physiological Society, 1987), 373–417.

7. ibid., 374.

8. Much of this section is gleaned from the classic textbook: E. C. Crosby, T. Humphrey, and E. W. Lauer, *Correlative Anatomy of the Nervous System* (New York: Macmillan, 1962). For more contemporary examples, see P. Rakic and W. Singer, eds., *Neurobiology of Neocortex* (New York: John Wiley and Sons, 1988); G. M. Edelman, W. E. Gall, and W. M. Cowan, eds., *Dynamic Aspects of Neocortical Function* (New York: John Wiley and Sons, 1984).

9. Wernicke's area is defined differently by different workers. Although Wernicke did not include them in his classic definition, many contemporary workers incorporate Brodmann's areas 39 (angular gyrus) and 40 (supramarginal gyrus) in Wernicke's area. This is probably appropriate since a lesion in area 39 leads to alexia (inability to read) and patients with damage to area 40 show a profound loss regarding the symbolism of language. For an entertaining discussion of the location of Wernicke's area, see J. E. Bogen and G. M. Bogen, "Wernicke's region—Where is it?" *Annals of New York Academy of Science* 280 (1976):834–43.

10. Positron emission tomographic (PET) studies reveal that semantic associations for words are processed in Brodmann's area 47 rather than in classic Broca's area (consisting of Brodmann's areas 44 and 45). Because of this, Petersen et al. think that classic Broca's area is not related to language-specific output programming but, instead, has general motor functions. See S. E. Petersen, P. T. Fox, M. I. Posner, M. Mintum, and M. E. Raichle, "Positron emission tomographic studies of the cortical anatomy of single-word processing," *Nature* 331 (1988):585–89.

11. A. Kendon, "Gesticulation and speech: Two aspects of the process of utterance," in M. R. Key, ed., *Nonverbal Communication and Language* (The Hague: Mouton, 1980), 207–27; see pp. 208–9.

12. Adam Kendon, "Human Gesture." Paper presented at the Wenner-Gren International Symposium on Tools, Language and Intelligence: Evolutionary Implications, Cascais, Portugal (1990).

13. S. Goldin-Meadow and H. Feldman, "The development of language-like communication without a language model," *Science* 197 (1977):401–3. S. Goldin-Meadow and C. Mylander, "Levels of structure in a language developed without a language model," in K. Gibson and A. Peterson, eds., *The Brain and Behavioral Development: Biosocial Dimensions* (New York: Aldine de Gruyter, 1989), 315–44.

14. Below is the transcription of a conversation that I had with Cynthea that gets at some of the thinking that underlies tap dancing. It also shows that the ability to tap dance is one of the better things about our species.

Q. One of the things I've noticed is that the way you teach a complicated tap step, say like the timestep, is that you break it apart. Or break it down as you say, so that we learn it by first learning the individual parts and then glue them together.
Cynthea: Right, so that they flow eventually.

Q. And you glue them together in short segments and then glue those short segments together into longer segments. And so it flows and it gets to the point where, I mean at first I couldn't do a timestep, but then I got to the point where all I have to do is think "timestep" and I can do a whole timestep. Is that the normal process?
Cynthea: That's how I was taught. So that for the memory, once you learn brush-hop for instance, you do that over again. Brush-hop, brush-hop. That enters the brain, it enters the body, it has to enter down to the feet, the knees.

Q. As one unit?
Cynthea: As one unit. Then you have to just go on. An extra shuffle-step. OK. It's a memory; it would be like memorizing a complete sentence. So then I go back and I say, "OK. Now it's brush-hop, second part shuffle-step."

Q. When you're dancing what are you thinking?
Cynthea: Early on, when performing, I would be thinking more of the counts or of the steps. Now, after performing for years, I'm able to just listen to the music. The memory is now developed, as with most dancers after a period of time, so that I don't have to think about what comes next. Sometimes in a piece I'll have to be aware if there's a space problem, where I have to cross somebody. That breaks my listening to the music and all of a sudden I have to say, "Oh, where is she? Am I going to miss her?" But otherwise I just listen to the music.

Q. Is that a larger extension of what we were just talking about? Is that "brush-hop, shuffle-step" but throughout the whole thing? Where you've got it down as one flowing—
Cynthea: Right, it's almost as if your brain is a computer and it's there. A lot of people say to musicians, "How could somebody who's playing a concert, say a Bach concert, do it without reading music?" You should never go to a concert and see somebody reading the music. The musician should know the music. Sometimes the music's there in front of him just to refer to in case there's a lapse of memory, but a concert pianist should be able to sit down and play a whole sonata. It's the same process, it's just part of him.

Q. So you actually just listen to the music as you're performing, and that's it. . . . What about choreography?
Cynthea: In choreographing, which is still new to me, the music usually comes first. If I close my eyes, I will see the steps or I will see the pattern or the next place it should go.

Q. Then would you say dance is a visual art?
Cynthea: Oh, it's very visual. It's all lines, although many dancers don't even understand that. It's as if each move is a word and you're telling something, whether it's a literal story or not. A lot of dancers don't even realize that it's the lines they're making, and the connecting of the lines.

Q. How do you prepare for a performance?
Cynthea: Before a concert, I will not physically go through every move. The better thing for me to do, and I think a lot of artists will tell you this, is almost like meditating. I close my eyes, and I go through every move in a piece. I'm hearing the music, and I can feel

and see my body go through every move. I know where my hands are, where my fingers are, where my head is, where my neck is.

Q. And do you experience it; do you actually feel as if you're doing it?
Cynthea: Yes, although in a sense I'm removed from it. It's almost as if I'm watching somebody on television doing it, in the sense of seeing it, but the feeling of it—

Q. When you watch a performance, are you at some level participating?
Cynthea: A really good dancer, yes. Somebody like Makarova, for instance, whose technique is so incredible that she's beyond her technique. The technique is there and you don't even think she's not going to make something or miss something. And she's so musical that she's able to take it beyond that and make one feel her moves. But only very few dancers do that. Astaire did that.

Q. Do you dream about dance or moving?
Cynthea: Not so much anymore. But I used to have a dream when I was a child. I would see myself fly in a grand jeté. A grand jeté is a big jump and everybody knows it when they see it. It's in every ballet. That was a wonderful dream. I would be in the grand jeté position and would go to take the jump and would just keep continuing, and I would go around the room and was definitely above looking down. That was the flight thing, you know. Now later on, as years have gone by, I've lost that. I was never to regain that space.

Q. What about the mental aspects of training?
Cynthea: That's very important. When I teach my professionals who have studied at very good schools, and we're going to do pirouettes, there's no reason why three pirouettes should mean anything to them. It should have evolved by now, and they're still getting caught up in two pirouettes. Now that is a block. Somewhere there was too much technique taught and they've lost the feeling of what it's like to turn. So the thing I point out to them, even in balances, is that you can't let your mind get in the way. You just simply do it. In other words, if you're going to take your hand off the bar and try to balance and you're thinking of all these things and your mind is overworking, you're not just going for it. And a lot of it is just simply, "This is where I have to be and this is where I'm going to be." So a lot of times the mind stops a natural movement.

Q. Are dancers getting better all the time? Is there an evolution of dance?

Cynthea: Well, when you look at old clips of people like Anna Pavlova, she was inspiring but certainly technically not anywhere up to where a dancer in a class would be today. The bodies have evolved and the feet and the backs and everything. People can do a lot more physically now than they did then. It doesn't mean that spiritually they've evolved to make the art form greater. I'm sure that if you saw Anna Pavlova dance and you saw somebody today dance, you might say that Pavlova was actually more inspirational than this other dancer who had her leg up to her nose and feet like this and had a back that went on for days and could turn maybe six times compared to Anna Pavlova's two turns. So it's a very individual thing. But certainly the physicalness has evolved. The kids on the street, look what they do: turning on their heads and their elbows!

4: Of Family Trees, Darwin's Theory, and the Origins of Bipedalism

1. Specifically, changes in the frequencies of alternate kinds of genes cause generations to change over time. For example, if eye color were controlled by two types of the eye-color gene (one for brown and one for blue), a population in which 95 percent of the eye genes were the blue type would look considerably different than a population in which 95 percent were the brown type. Thus, although the ingredients would be the same within the two groups, the relative amounts of the different types of eye-color gene would cause the populations to appear generally different (but with overlap) as far as eye color goes. In this sense, evolution can simply be viewed as a change in gene frequencies over time.

2. So much for the lighter side of Malthus. What one doesn't read in most textbooks on evolutionary theory are Malthus's proposals for restraining human population growth in *An Essay on the Principle of Population* (New York: W. W. Norton & Co., 1976.) He suggested that the poor were having too many children and that the laws that protected poor children from starvation (i.e., that gave them the right to parish assistance) should be abolished. He further proposed that the lower classes should be instructed that it would

229

be immoral for a man to marry and bear children unless he knows he can support his family. If a poor man chose to marry anyway, "All parish assistance should be denied him; and he should be left to the uncertain support of private charity. He should be taught to know that the laws of nature, which are the laws of God, had doomed him and his family to suffer for disobeying their repeated admonitions; that he had no claim of right on society for the smallest portion of food. . . ." (135–36). This was controversial stuff even in Malthus's day. Jonathan Swift's satirical *Modest Proposal for Preventing the Children of Poor People from being a Burden to their Parents or the Country* was perhaps the most famous retort to Malthus's essay. Swift wickedly suggested that Irish babies should be fattened to make food for the rich.

3. Some workers put the date of the CA at six or seven million years ago, others place it at four or five. For simplicity's sake, I accept five million years ago as a reasonable approximation.

4. The arboreal theory was elaborated by Elliot Smith and F. Wood Jones early in this century. See Jones's book *Arboreal Man* (E. Arnold, 1916). More recently, Matt Cartmill, "Rethinking primate origins," *Science* 184 (1974):436–43, has emphasized the importance of general primate adaptations for catching insects. His "bug-snatching" theory puts a new twist on the arboreal theory.

5. See A. Zihlmann, "Pygmy chimps, people, and the pundits," *New Scientist,* 15 November 1984, 39–40.

6. The last word on the knuckle-walking debate is not yet in. The third great ape, the orangutan, is not a knuckle-walker. Orangutans are from Asia and more distantly related to humans than the gorilla or chimpanzee. They lack the bony signs of knuckle-walking for the simple reason that they do not engage in it. In fact, orangutans spend as little time as possible on the ground. When they are on the ground, however, orangutans rest and move on their fists or palms rather than their knuckles. Although orangutans are not knuckle-walkers, it is extremely interesting that all three of the great apes ball their hands up in one way or another when moving on the ground. Perhaps this tendency was inherited from their common ancestor.

7. M. D. Leakey, "Pliocene footprints at Laetoli, northern Tanzania,"

Antiquity 52 (1978):133. See also M. D. Leakey and R. L. Hay, "Pliocene footprints in the Laetoli Beds at Laetoli, northern Tanzania," *Nature* 278 (1979):317–23.

8. R. H. Tuttle, "Kinesiological inferences and evolutionary implications from Laetoli bipedal trails G-1, G-2/3, and A," in M. D. Leakey and J. M. Harris, eds., *Laetoli, A Pliocene Site In Northern Tanzania* (Oxford: Clarendon Press, 1987), 503–23.

9. Though controversial, Tuttle's work is so thorough and he has answered his critics so skillfully that he's convinced me that the toe bones that made the Laetoli impressions were probably flat rather than curved.

10. S. L. Washburn, "Tools and human evolution," *Scientific American* 203 (1960):63–75.

11. This notion of different parts of the body evolving at different rates is called "mosaic evolution."

12. In fact, Sherwood Washburn's name is linked with both theories.

13. A number of anthropologists now support this idea, which was suggested by S. Linton, "Woman the gatherer: Male bias in anthropology," in W. Jacobs, ed., *Women in Cross-Cultural Perspective* (Champaign-Urbana: University of Illinois Press, 1971), 9–21.

14. C. Boesch and H. Boesch, "Possible causes of sex differences in the use of natural hammers by wild chimpanzees," *Journal of Human Evolution* 13 (1984):415–40.

15. P. Shipman, "Scavenging or hunting in early hominids: Theoretical framework and tests," *American Anthropologist* 88 (1986):27–43.

16. C. O. Lovejoy, "The origin of man," *Science* 211 (1981):341–50.

17. A. L. Zihlman, "Gathering stories for hunting human nature: A review essay," *Feminist Studies* 11 (1985):365–77.

18. ibid., 374. On p. 346 of Lovejoy, "Origin" (see note 16, chapter 4), Lovejoy says: "Human females are continually sexually receptive (79). . . ." Footnote 79 (p. 350) reads: "D. C. Johanson, personal communication."

19. N. M. Tanner, "Gathering by females: The chimpanzee model revisited and the gathering hypothesis," in W. G. Kinzey, ed., *The*

Evolution of Human Behavior: Primate Models (State University of New York Press, 1987), 3–27; see pp. 14, 18.

20. J. Goodall, *The Chimpanzees of Gombe* (Cambridge: Belknap Press, 1986), 145.

21. Whenever I read about the large size of human penises compared with those of other mammals, I am transported back to an experience I had in 1979 while doing research at the Smithsonian. I entered a spacious room that contained various alcohol-preserved specimens and began to search the shelves for the primate brains. As I peered into one jar, I thought "that looks like a—no, it couldn't be." When I looked at the next jar, I thought "Why that also looks like a—Nooo." Along about the third jar, I realized that, indeed, I had happened upon a collection of preserved penises. I must admit that I then observed the entire collection with some awe. What marvelous variety there is in this most fundamental of animal appendages!

    According to William G. Eberhard, a leading expert on animal genitalia in *Sexual Selection and Animal Genitalia* (Cambridge: Harvard University Press, 1985), the most likely selective factor explaining large penis size in humans is tactile stimulation of the female. Apparently, the cervix of the human female actually withdraws from the opening of the vagina during sexual arousal. However, sensory stimuli from a protruded glans of the human penis can trigger contraction of the female reproductive tract that results in sperm transport, thereby increasing the likelihood of conception. Thus, sexual selection by females for males that were adept at sexual stimulation may have been a contributing factor to large penis size in males.

22. A. R. E. Sinclair, M. D. Leakey, and M. Norton-Griffiths, "Migration and hominid bipedalism," *Nature* 324 (1987):307–8.

23. P. E. Wheeler, "Stand tall and stay cool," *New Scientist*, 12 May 1988, 62–65.

24. P. E. Wheeler, "The loss of functional body hair in man: The influence of thermal environment, body form and bipedality." *Journal of Human Evolution* 14 (1985):23–28. Also see P. E. Wheeler, "The evolution of bipedality and loss of functional body hair in hominids," *Journal of Human Evolution* 13 (1984):91–98.

25. R. W. Wrangham, "The significance of African apes for reconstructing human social evolution," in *The Evolution of Human Behavior: Primate Models,* ed. W. G. Kinzey (State University of New York Press, 1987), 51–71.

26. G. Richards, "Freed hands or enslaved feet? A note on the behavioural implications of ground-dwelling bipedalism," *Journal of Human Evolution* 15 (1986):143–50; see p. 146.

27. As this book goes to press, reports are circulating that additional fragmentary fossils representing *Australopithecus afarensis* have recently been recovered from Ethiopia. It is rumored that these fossils may be older than the previously discovered Hadar (or Laetoli) specimens.

5: Boy Brain, Girl Brain

1. Sperry's Nobel Prize was shared with David Hubel and Torsten Wiesel who did pioneering work on brain structures involved in the visual system.

2. R. W. Sperry, "Mental unity following surgical disconnection of the cerebral hemispheres," in *The Harvey Lecture Series,* vol. 62 (New York: Academic Press, 1968).

3. R. W. Sperry, "Consciousness, personal identity, and the divided brain." Public lecture presented at the Smithsonian Institution, 1977. Also in D. F. Benson and E. Zaidel, eds., *The Dual Brain* (New York: The Guilford Press, 1985), 11–26; see p. 17.

4. For a review of these and other techniques, see S. Springer and G. Deutsch, *Left Brain, Right Brain* (New York: W. H. Freeman and Co., 1989) and J. McGlone, "Sex differences in human brain asymmetry: A critical survey," *Behavioral and Brain Sciences* 3 (1980):215–63.

5. For a review, see D. Falk, "Brain lateralization in primates and its evolution in hominids," *Yearbook of Physical Anthropology* 30 (1987):107–25.

6. For details, see N. Geschwind and A. M. Galaburda, *Cerebral La-*

teralization: Biological Mechanisms, Associations, and Pathology (Cambridge: MIT Press, 1987).

7. For examples, see M. S. Gazzaniga and J. E. LeDoux, *The Integrated Mind* (New York: Plenum Press, 1978).

8. J. E. Bogen, concluding overview in A. G. Reeves, ed., *Epilepsy and the Corpus Callosum* (New York: Plenum Press, 1985), 515–24; see p. 518.

9. S. M. Ferguson, M. Rayport, and W. S. Corrie, "Neuropsychiatric observations on behavioral consequences of corpus callosum section for seizure control." In Reeves (note 8, chapter 5), 501–14; see p. 504.

10. For discussion, see Sperry (note 3, chapter 5).

11. A number of studies report different lateralization patterns for musicians and nonmusicians, and there is some evidence that musically sophisticated listeners utilize their left hemispheres to recognize the melody. This literature is reviewed in Falk, "Brain lateralization" (note 5, chapter 5).

12. Sperry (note 3, chapter 5), 23.

13. J. S. Hyde and M. C. Linn, "Gender differences in verbal ability: A meta-analysis," *Psychological Bulletin* 104 (1988):53–69. However, the authors conclude that these statistically significant results are of no practical significance.

14. J. Hyde, E. Fennema, and S. J. Lamon, "Gender differences in mathematics performance: A meta-analysis," *Psychological Bulletin* 107 (1990):139–55.

15. Reviewed in Falk, "Brain lateralization" (note 5, chapter 5).

16. This figure was provided courtesy of Roland Guay. For more information, see R. Guay and E. McDaniel, "Correlates of performance on spatial aptitude tests," Final Report grant No. DAHC 19-77-G-0019 (Alexandria, Va.: U. S. Army Research Institute for the Behavior and Social Sciences, 1978). The answer to the task is B.

17. For further discussion of these differences, see M. Hines, "Gonadal hormones and human cognitive development," in *Hormones, Brains, and Behaviour,* ed. J. Balthazart, *Comparative Physiology*

8:51–63. See also L. S. Allen, M. Hines, J. E. Shryne, and R. A. Gorski, "Two sexually dimorphic cell groups in the human brain," *The Journal of Neuroscience* 9 (1989):497–506. For a while, it was believed that certain measurements of another area of the brain, the corpus callosum, were larger in females than males. However, numerous workers were unable to replicate this finding and it is now questionable whether significant sex differences in callosal anatomy exist. For an excellent review, see S. F. Witelson and D. L Kigar, "Neuroanatomical aspects of hemisphere specialization in humans," in *Duality and Unity Of The Brain*, ed. D. Ottoson. Proceedings of an International Symposium at the Wenner-Gren Center, Stockholm, May 29–31, 1986 (New York: Macmillan, 1987), 466–95.

18. J. McGlone (note 4, chapter 5).

19. D. Kimura, "Sex differences in cerebral organization for speech and praxic functions," *Canadian Journal of Psychology* 37 (1983):19–35; D. Kimura and R. A. Harshman, "Sex differences in brain organization for verbal and nonverbal functions," *Progress in Brain Research* 61 (1984):423–41. See, however, another study that presents evidence against an intrahemispheric sex difference: A. Kertesz and T. Benke, "Sex equality in intrahemispheric language organization," *Brain and Language* 37 (1989):401–8.

20. For information about petalias see M. LeMay, "Morphological cerebral asymmetries of modern man, fossil man, and nonhuman primates," *Annals of the New York Academy of Sciences* 280 (1976):349–60; A. M. Galaburda, M. LeMay, T. L. Kemper and N. Geschwind, "Right-left asymmetries in the brain," *Science* 199 (1978):852–56. LeMay's findings were confirmed by D. Bear, D. Schiff, J. Saver, M. Greenberg, and R. Freeman, "Quantitative analysis of cerebral asymmetries," *Archives of Neurology* 43 (1986):598–603. The finding of more reversals in the pattern of petalias for women by Bear and his colleagues is in keeping with still another study that reported more reversals for women from the normal pattern of a longer left temporal plane: J. A. Wada, R. Clark and A. Hamm, "Cerebral hemisphere asymmetry in humans," *Archives of Neurology* 32 (1975):239–46.

21. Kimura and Hampson reported their findings at the November 1988 meeting of the Society for Neurosciences, in Toronto. See E.

Hampson and D. Kimura, "Reciprocal effects of hormonal fluctuations on human motor and perceptual-spatial skills," *Behavioral Neuroscience* 102 (1988):456–59.

22. S. A. Berenbaum and M. Hines, "Hormonal influences on sex-typed toy preferences." Paper presented to the Society for Research in Child Development (Kansas City, Missouri, 1989).

23. Hines, (note 17, chapter 5), 51–63.

24. P. Flor-Henry, "Functional hemispheric asymmetry and psychopathology," *Integrated Psychiatry* 1 (1983):46–52.

25. D. Falk, L. Konigsberg, C. Helmkamp, J. Cheverud, M. Vannier, and C. Hildebolt, "Endocranial suture closure in rhesus macaques *(Macaca mulatta),*" *American Journal of Physical Anthropology* 80 (1989):417–28; L. Konigsberg, D. Falk, C. Hildebolt, M. Vannier, J. Cheverud, and C. Helmkamp, "External brain morphology in rhesus macaques *(Macaca mulatta),*" *Journal of Human Evolution* 19 (1990):269–84; A. Masters, D. Falk, and T. Gage, "Effects of age and gender on the location and orientation of the foramen magnum in rhesus macaques *(Macaca mulatta),*" *American Journal of Physical Anthropology* 86 (1991):75–80.

26. R. Weiss, "Women's skills linked to estrogen levels," *Science News* 134 (1988):341.

27. T. E. Robinson, J. B. Becker, D. M. Camp, and A. Mansour, "Variation in the pattern of behavioral and brain asymmetries due to sex differences," in S. D. Glick, ed., *Cerebral Lateralization in Nonhuman Species* (New York: Academic Press, 1985), 185–231; see p. 195.

28. Parts of this section will also be published in an edited volume from the 1990 Wenner-Gren International Symposium on Tools, Language and Intelligence: Evolutionary Implications, Kathleen Gibson and Tim Ingold, eds. (New York: Cambridge University Press).

29. S. J. C. Gaulin and R. W. FitzGerald, "Home-range size as a predictor of mating systems in *Microtus,*" *Journal of Mammalogy* 69 (1988):311–19; "Sexual selection for spatial-learning ability," *Animal Behavior* 37 (1989):322–31.

30. F. Nottebohm, "Asymmetries in neural control of vocalization in the canary," in S. Harnad, R. Doty, L. Goldstein, J. Jaynes, and G.

Krauthamer, eds., *Lateralization in the Nervous System* (New York: Academic Press, 1977), 23–44; "From bird song to neurogenesis," *Scientific American*, February 1989, 74–79.

31. For discussion, see D. Falk, C. Hildebolt, J. Cheverud, M. Vannier, R. C. Helmkamp, and L. Konigsberg, "Cortical asymmetries in frontal lobes of rhesus monkeys (*Macaca mulatta*)," *Brain Research* 512 (1990):40–45.

32. T. Wynn, *The Evolution of Spatial Competence*, (Champaign-Urbana: University of Illinois Press, 1989).

33. Two things to remember: (1) Genes that are selected for in one sex are extremely likely to affect the other, and (2) there is a huge amount of "overlap" in the abilities of males and females.

6: Lucy's Child: Mix-up at the Hospital

1. D. C. Johanson, "Ethiopia yields first 'family' of early man," *National Geographic* 150 (1976):790–811.

2. D. C. Johanson and M. Taieb, "Plio-Pleistocene hominid discoveries in Hadar, Ethiopia," *Nature* 260 (1976):293–97.

3. Museum specimens are typically given identifications that indicate the museum and/or location where they were found. Thus, KNM-ER stands for Kenya National Museums, East Rudolf; KNM-WT indicates the same museum but a West Turkana site; and OH means Olduvai Hominid.

4. For information regarding climate and habitat at Hadar, see R. Bonnefille, A. Vincens, and G. Buchet, "Palynology, stratigraphy and palaeoenvironment of a Pliocene hominid site (2.9–3.0 M.Y.) at Hadar, Ethiopia," *Palaeogeography, Palaeoclimatology, Palaeoecology* 60 (1987):249–81. For information about Laetoli, see R. Bonnefille and G. Riollet, "Palynological spectra from the upper Laetolil beds," in M. D. Leakey and J. M. Harris, eds., *Laetoli, A Pliocene Site in Northern Tanzania* (Oxford: Clarendon Press, 1987), 52–61.

5. *International Code of Zoological Nomenclature*, International Trust for Zoological Nomenclature, London, 2nd ed. (1964). (There is

now a third edition, 1985, of the Code, but the second edition was in use at the time *Australopithecus afarensis* was named.)

6. D. C. Johanson, T. D. White, and Y. Coppens, "A new species of the genus *Australopithecus* (Primates: Hominidae) from the Pliocene of eastern Africa," *Kirtlandia* 28 (1978):1–14; see p. 8.

7. N. T. Boaz, F. C. Howell, and M. L. McCrossin, "Faunal age of the Usno, Shungura B and Hadar Formations, Ethiopia," *Nature* 300 (1982):633–35.

8. D. C. Johanson and T. D. White, "A systematic assessment of early African hominids," *Science* 203 (1979):321–30.

9. For examples, see letters from M. H. Day, M. D. Leakey, and T. R. Olson; and from R. E. F. Leakey and A. Walker, "On the status of *Australopithecus afarensis*," *Science* 207 (1980):1102–3.

10. To give credit where it is due, Tobias first described the O/M sinus system in robust australopithecines in his classic monograph on *Zinjanthropus*. See P. V. Tobias, *Olduvai Gorge*, vol. 2 (New York: Cambridge University Press, 1967). Holloway was the first to note that an O/M sinus system is also present in the Hadar fossil material in R. L. Holloway, "The endocast of the Omo juvenile L338y-6 hominid specimen," *American Journal of Physical Anthropology* 54 (1981):109–18.

11. H. Browning, "The confluence of dural venous sinuses," *American Journal of Anatomy* 93 (1953):307–29.

12. D. Johanson and J. Shreeve, *Lucy's Child* (New York: William Morrow, 1989), 117.

13. For example, Kimbel and White's discussion of O/M sinuses in W. H. Kimbel and T. D. White, "Variation, sexual dimorphism and the taxonomy of *Australopithecus*," in F. Grine, ed., *Evolutionary History of the "Robust" Australopithecines* (New York: Plenum Press, 1988), 175–92, consisted of the following:
"Falk and Conroy's conclusions based on cranial venous flow patterns have been critically examined in other publications (Kimbel, 1984; Kimbel et al., 1985) and will not be addressed here." (186)
Turning to the 1985 publication that they cite above, W. H. Kimbel, T. C. White, and D. C. Johanson, "Craniodental morphol-

ogy of the hominids from Hadar and Laetoli: Evidence of *"Paranthropus"* and *Homo* in the mid-Pliocene for eastern Africa?" in E. Delson, ed., *Ancestors: The Hard Evidence* (New York: Alan R. Liss, 1985), 120–37, for their critical examination of the cranial blood flow evidence, we read:

"Detailed discussions of venous drainage patterns and their value for hominid phylogeny reconstruction are available elsewhere (Falk and Conroy, 1983; Kimbel, 1984) and are therefore not reiterated here." (36)

Finally, turning to the 1984 article they cite, Kimbel summed up the view from Johanson's camp but, contrary to the assertions quoted above, he did so without reference to, or discussion of, the evidence discussed by Conroy and me regarding cranial blood flow: W. H. Kimbel, "Variation in the pattern of cranial venous sinuses and hominid phylogeny," *American Journal of Physical Anthropology* 63(1984):243–63.

14. ibid., 243.

15. Johanson and Shreeve (note 12, chapter 6), 122

16. Actually, the specimen was discovered in 1985, but the discovery was not published until 1986 (see next note).

17. A. Walker, R. E. Leakey, J. M. Harris, and F. H. Brown, "2.5-Myr *Australopithecus boisei* from west of Lake Turkana, Kenya," *Nature* 322 (1986):517–22.

18. See D. Falk, "Hominid evolution (letter)," *Science* 234 (1986):11.

19. For a wonderfully written review article, read R. H. Tuttle, "What's new in African paleoanthropology?" *Annual Review of Anthropology* 17 (1988):391–426; see p. 397.

20. R. R. Skelton, H. M. McHenry, and G. M. Drawhorn, "Phylogenetic analysis of early hominids," *Current Anthropology* 27 (1986): 21–43.

21. F. C. Howell, Foreword, in F. Grine, ed., *Evolutionary History of the "Robust" Australopithecines* (New York: Aldine de Gruyter, 1988), xii.

22. L. S. B. Leakey, P. V. Tobias, and J. R. Napier, "A new species of the genus *Homo* from Olduvai Gorge," *Nature* 202 (1964):7–10.

23. F. Brown, J. Harris, R. Leakey, and A. Walker, "Early *Homo erectus* skeleton from west Lake Turkana, Kenya," *Nature* 316 (1985): 788–92.

24. D. C. Johanson, F. T. Masao, G. G. Eck, T. D. White, R. C. Walter, W. H. Kimbel, B. Asfaw, P. Manega, P. Ndessokia, and G. Suwa, "New partial skeleton of *Homo habilis* from Olduvai Gorge, Tanzania," *Nature* 327 (1987):205–9.

25. ibid., 209

7: The Radiator Theory of Brain Evolution

1. Whenever possible, presence or absence of the posterior condyloid, mastoid, occipital, and parietal foramina were determined. I also observed whether or not hypoglossal canals were single or divided and, of course, if an enlarged O/M sinus was present or absent. My raw data and analysis can be found in D. Falk, "Evolution of cranial blood drainage in hominids: Enlarged occipital/marginal sinuses and emissary foramina," *American Journal of Physical Anthropology* 70 (1986):311–24.

2. An earlier, stimulating study by G. I. Boyd showed that emissary foramina occurred in much lower frequencies in apes than in humans: "The emissary foramina of the cranium in man and the anthropoids," *Journal of Anatomy* 65 (1930):108–21. Boyd's study was influential in my decision to pursue emissary foramina in the hominid fossil record. Sometimes there's gold in old, nearly forgotten journal articles!

3. M. A. Baker, "A brain-cooling system in mammals," *Scientific American* 240 (1979):130–39; see p. 136.

4. M. Cabanac and H. Brinnel, "Blood flow in the emissary veins of the human head during hyperthermia," *European Journal of Applied Physiology* 54 (1985): 172–76.

5. See target article and open peer commentary: D. Falk, "Brain evolution in *Homo*: The "radiator" theory," *Behavioral and Brain Sciences* 13 (1990):333–81.

6. A. L. Zihlman and B. A. Cohn, "Responses of hominid skin to the savanna," *Suid-Afrikaase Tydskrif vir Wetenskap* 82 (1986):89–90; "The adaptive response of human skin to the savanna," *Human Evolution* 3 (1988):397–409.

7. The circumstances under which *Homo erectus* gave rise to *Homo sapiens*, once again, pits some (but not all) paleoanthropologists against molecular geneticists (see Chapter 3). Molecular evidence based on comparative studies of mitochondrial DNA (which is located outside of the nuclei of cells, and is inherited solely through the maternal line) suggests to some that all living people are descended from one woman who lived in Africa a mere 200,000 years ago (this is known as the Eve hypothesis). Presumably, the group of early *Homo sapiens* to which Eve belonged migrated out of Africa, colonized the world, and thoroughly out-competed the other hominids who already occupied these newly colonized areas. (To give credit where it is due, this idea was proposed ten years ago in the "out of Africa" theory of paleontologist Christopher Stringer.) However, if the Eve hypothesis were true it would mean that much of the known fossil record represents individuals who became extinct without leaving offspring, which seems counter-intuitive to many critics. Numerous paleoanthropologists, therefore, reject the Eve hypothesis, which they say is based on false assumptions about the mutation rate of mitochondrial DNA, as well as on a disregard for mitochondrial DNA's possible role as a subject for natural selection. They also believe that if it were properly calibrated, the mitochondrial clock would be shown to actually measure the migration of *Homo erectus* out of Africa (at least one million years ago), rather than the more recent dispersal of *Homo sapiens*. Paleoanthropologists who reject the Eve hypothesis believe that *Homo sapiens* emerged simultaneously in various parts of the world, a process C. Loring Brace calls "in situ continuity." See his discussion in C. L. Brace, "Tales of the phylogenetic woods: The evolution and significance of evolutionary trees," *American Journal of Physical Anthropology* 56 (1981): 411–29. According to Brace, the one trend that characterized the transformation of earlier hominids into modern humans was reduction in robusticity of bones and teeth. He attributes the simultaneous emergence of *Homo* in various regions to reduced selection for large (strong) bodies and teeth that occurred in conjunction with the rapid spread of hunting and culinary technology.

The interested reader is referred to C. L. Brace, *The Stages of Human Evolution*, 4th ed. (Englewood Cliffs, N.J.: Prentice-Hall, 1991).

8. C. B. Stringer and R. Grün, "Time for the last Neandertals," *Nature* 351 (1991):701–2.

9. J. E. Pfeiffer, *The Creative Explosion* (New York: Harper and Row, 1982). For a different view, see C. B. Stringer, "The emergence of modern humans," *Scientific American*, December 1990:98–104.

8: Braindance

1. K. Zilles, E. Armstrong, A. Schleicher, and H.-J. Kretschmann, "The human pattern of gyrification in the cerebral cortex," *Anatomy and Embryology* 179 (1988):173–79.

2. A. B. Scheibel, L. A. Paul, I. Fried, A. B. Forsythe, U. Tomiyasu, A. Wechsler, A. Kao, and J. Slotnick, "Dendritic organization of the anterior speech area," *Experimental Neurology* 87 (1985):109–17.

3. R. E. Passingham, "The brain and intelligence," *Brain Behavior and Evolution* 11 (1975):1–15.

4. My friend, William Calvin, has a somewhat different theory about the evolution of neurological sequencers, which he believes resulted from selection for throwing ability. Read his wonderful *The Throwing Madonna: Essays on the Brain* (New York: McGraw-Hill, 1983).

5. J. D. Maser and G. G. Gallup, "Theism as a by-product of natural selection," *Journal of Religion* 70 (1990):515–32.

6. W. Kohler, *The Mentality of Apes* (London: Routledge and Kegan Paul, 1925; New York: Liveright, 1976), 145 of 1976 ed.

7. Maser and Gallup (note 5, chapter 8), 14.

8. ibid., 19.

9. However, not everyone agrees with his interpretation, as shown by P. G. Bahn, "Eating people is wrong," *Nature* 348 (1990):395. In fact, interpretation of evidence that is theoretically associated with

cannibalism in the fossil record is one of those controversial topics that has as many naysayers as advocates.

10. D. R. Harris, "Aboriginal subsistence in a tropical rain forest environment: food procurement, cannibalism, and population regulation in northeastern Australia," in M. Harris and E. B. Ross, eds., *Food and Evolution* (Philadelphia: Temple University Press, 1987), 357–85; see p. 372.

11. D. Falk, "Implications of the evolution of writing for the origin of language: Can a paleoneurologist find happiness in the Neolithic?" Proceedings of NATO Advanced Study Institute, in B. Chiarelli, P. Lieberman, and J. Wind, eds., *The Origins of Human Language* (The Netherlands: Kluwer Academic Press, in press), 1991.

12. D. Schmandt-Besserat, "The earliest precursor of writing," *Scientific American* 238 (1978):51–59; "Oneness, twoness, threeness; How ancient accountants invented numbers," *The Sciences* 20 (1987):44–48.

13. See also Alexander Marshack's discussion about Paleolithic art: A. Marshack, "Hierarchical Evolution of the Human Capacity: The Paleolithic Evidence." Fifty-fourth James Arthur Lecture on the Evolution of the Human Brain, American Museum of Natural History, New York, 1985.

14. R. Lewin, *In the Age of Mankind* (Washington, D.C.: Smithsonian Books, 1988), 142–43.

15. The urgency of these issues is underscored in an important article by P. R. Ehrlich and E. O. Wilson (*Science* 253 [1991]:758–62): Almost 40 percent of all the food supply for all land animals and decomposers is "used, coopted, or forgone" because of *Homo sapiens*. This is causing an alarming rate of extinction of species that live on land. Furthermore, since the human population is expected to double in the next fifty years (to over ten billion people), a five- to tenfold increase in global economic activity will be required to meet human needs. The authors conclude that, "The indispensable strategy for saving our fellow living creatures and ourselves in the long run, is, as the evidence compellingly shows, to reduce the scale of human activities. The task of accomplishing this goal will involve a cooperative worldwide effort unprecedented in history.

Unless humanity can move determinedly in that direction, all of the efforts now going into in situ conservation, will eventually lead no-where, and our descendants' future will be at risk" (761).

16. E. Armstrong, "The limbic system and culture," *Human Nature* 2 (1991):117–36; E. Armstrong, M. R. Clarke, E. M. Hill, "Relative size of the anterior thalamic nuclei differentiates anthropoids by social system," *Brain, Behavior and Evolution* 30 (1987):263–71.

9: Brainwar

1. Provided by Lauren Gage, age six years.

2. For an excellent treatment, see Meredith Small, ed., *Female Primates: Studies by Women Primatologists* (New York: Alan R. Liss, 1984). Jane Lancaster's Introduction is especially insightful.

3. Sarah Blaffer Hrdy is responsible for this idea. It is unfortunate that her work is frequently excluded from women's studies. Read *The Woman That Never Evolved* (Cambridge: Harvard University Press, 1981).

4. Much of the information in this section is taken from Goodall's wonderful volume, *The Chimpanzees of Gombe, Patterns of Behavior* (Cambridge: Belknap Press, 1986).

5. ibid., 272.

6. F. de Waal, *Peacemaking Among Primates* (Cambridge: Harvard University Press, 1989).

7. ibid., 65–66.

8. ibid., 238–39.

9. As I write this sentence, I hear a "Yeah, but" from the cultural determinists! True, the other species of chimpanzee, bonobos or pygmy chimps, has been noted for its remarkable gentleness. However, as de Waal points out on page 221 of his book (note 6, chapter 9) this same opinion prevailed about common chimpanzees until a decade ago. Pygmy chimpanzees have, as yet, barely been studied. Furthermore, de Waal notes that an astonishing number of bonobos

lack fingers, toes, or hands, and he suggests that this may be linked with aggression.

10. B. M. Knauft, "Reconsidering violence in simple human societies," *Current Anthropology* 28 (1987):457–500.

11. ibid., 466.

12. At the 1986 business meeting of the American Anthropological Association (AAA), members unanimously passed a proposed resolution endorsing the Seville Statement on Violence. The Seville Statement was drafted by a committee of scientists from various disciplines and nations at a meeting on May 16, 1986 that was sponsored by the Spanish National UNESCO Commission. The text of the AAA resolution read in part:

The propositions are: (1) It is scientifically incorrect to say that we have inherited a tendency to make war from our animal ancestors. (2) It is scientifically incorrect to say that war or any other violent behavior is genetically programmed into our human nature. (3) It is scientifically incorrect to say that in the course of human evolution there has been a selection for aggressive behavior more than for other kinds of behavior. (4) It is scientifically incorrect to say that humans have a "violent brain." (5) It is scientifically incorrect to say that war is caused by "instinct" or any other single motivation. The Statement on Violence concludes that humanity is not condemned to war by biology, but to the contrary, humanity is capable of investing peace, as well as war.

Because of widespread pessimism about the possibilities of reducing interpersonal violence and/or implementing nonviolent alternatives to war, the Statement on Violence merits wide circulation and discussion. Anthropologists and others are requested to reflect upon how they might use, or expand upon, the Statement on Violence in their various roles as teachers, researchers, consultants, and citizens.

Subsequently, the resolution was submitted to a mail ballot of the full AAA membership, where it passed. Although the resolution was clearly well intended, I voted against it because Proposition 1 is probably false, and propositions 2 through 4 have not yet been tested sufficiently to permit specific statements about what is or is not scientifically incorrect. (Proposition 5, however, appears valid.)

However, the AAA resolution reflects current thinking among social anthropologists, namely an abhorrence of the possibility that our species might be biologically predisposed for aggression. Of course, many biological anthropologists (including this one) suspect otherwise. If we are right, no amount of resolving or asserting is going to change matters. On the other hand, understanding and dealing directly with the truth might. Ironically, this paradigmatic difference between subdisciplines of anthropology has itself had a long history of stimulating aggressive and emotional academic exchanges. Although the topic of nature versus nurture is a touchy one for anthropologists and for other social scientists, it is, of course, based largely on a false dichotomy. For humans, there can be no nature without nurture, nor nurture without nature. Both are crucial, and it is just plain silly to argue otherwise.

13. M. Daly and M. Wilson, *Homicide* (New York: Aldine de Gruyter, 1988).

14. ibid., 24.

15. ibid., 128.

16. Although this section reads like science fiction, it's not. Much of its content is taken from an August 7, 1989, *U.S. News and World Report* cover story, "America's Doomsday Project," by Stevan Emerson.

17. The information presented here is taken from an article by Robert C. Toth of the *Los Angeles Times*, that was published in the July 23, 1989 issue of the *Sunday Times Union*, in Albany, New York.

18. This information is from a *Los Angeles Times* article that was published in the *Sunday Times Union* in Albany, New York, on February 11, 1990.

19. However, at least one military expert, Col. Harry G. Summers, Jr., argues that "the nuclear era is over" ("How to be the world's policeman," *The New York Times Magazine*, 19 May 1991:40–46). He claims that nuclear weapons are not weapons of war but, instead, are useful only for deterrence against their use by other powers. Since deterrence does not require the "thousands upon thousands

of warheads now stockpiled by the superpowers," Summers reasons that the number of nuclear weapons will be greatly reduced and hence so will their threat. Summers also believes that the United States' conventional forces should be bolstered. Despite his optimism about the nonthreat of nuclear weapons, Summers acknowledges that the following nine countries now have them: the United States, Soviet Union, China, Britain, France, India, Israel, Pakistan, and South Africa.

20. The United States House of Representatives declined a wise investment when it voted to eliminate all funding for the search for extraterrestrial intelligence (SETI) from NASA's 1991 budget. Fortunately, these funds were subsequently restored. According to a report by Richard Kerr in *Nature* 249 (1990):249–50, the technology now exists to develop an instrument that could monitor 20 million radio channels every second, and for a "relatively cheap price tag" at that. Although admittedly it's a long shot, confirmation of a "them" out there would not hurt the cause of terrestrial unification.

21. Goodall (note 4, chapter 9), 534.

Index

Abri Blanchard, France, 185
Afterlife, 181, 183
Aggression, 7–8, 199–220
  in apes, 200–211, 244–245
  in chimpanzees, 25, 200–201,
    204–211
  homicide, 212–216
  patrolling, 210–211, 216–219
AL 122-28, 36–37
Allometric scaling, 43, 46
Ambition, 180
American Anthropological Associa-
    tion, 245–246
*American Journal of Physical Anthro-
    pology*, 43, 131
American Sign Language for the Deaf,
    54
Amphetamines, 117–118
Anterior thalamic nucleus, 196, 197
Anthropoids, brain lateralization in,
    122
Anwander, Walter, 156, 159

Apes:
  aggression among, 25, 200–211,
    244–245
  family tree of, 77–78
  O/M sinuses in, 154
  *See also specific types of apes,
    e.g.* Bonobos; Chimpanzees;
    Gorillas
Aphasia, 110
Arapesh of New Guinea, 200
Arboreal theory, 80–81, 230
Arboreal vestiges, 97–99
Ardrey, Robert, 199–200
Arm bones of australopithecines, 14,
    150, 166
Armstrong, Este, 47, 48, 178, 196,
    197
Arnhem Zoo, 209-10
Art, 6, 173, 184, 188–193
Association areas of the brain, 66–68,
    176, 177
  linkage with sensory areas, 62

249

Association areas of the brain *(cont'd)*
  prefrontal association cortex, 63–
    66, 176, 177, 180
Attention, 64
Auditory abilities, *see* Hearing
Auditory association cortex, 62
Australian aborigines, 182
Australopithecines, 139
  arm bones of, 14, 150
  Australopithecus afarensis, see Aus-
    tralopithecus afarensis
  bipedalism, *see* Bipedalism
  brain size of, 32, 76, 163
  cerebral cortex of, 4
  cognitive abilities of, 76
  dentition, 13, 14, 18, 26
  derivation of name, 11
  first discovered fossil, *see* Taung
    fossil
  gracile, *see* Gracile australopithe-
    cines
  Homo, characteristics distinguished
    from, 145, 169–170
  life-style of, 25–28
  proponents of apelike features of, 2,
    4, 13–14, 33, 46–48
  proponents of humanlike features
    of, 2, 4, 10, 12–13, 32–34,
    47–48
    historical reasons for, 12, 21
    lamboid suture vs. lunate sulcus
      controversy, 33–37
    Taung fossil is child and, 12–13
  rate of development, 14
  robust, *see* Robust australopithe-
    cines
  types of, 15–21, 139
Australopithecus afarensis, 128, 167,
  233
  as ancestral to robust australopithe-
    cines, 135, 137
  on family tree, 167
  naming of, 130, 131
  variations in, 129, 131, 142, 143
Australopithecus africanus:
  as gracile australopithecines, *see*
    Gracile australopithecines

origin of the name, 12, 13
"Australopithecus, Homo erectus,
  and the single species hypothesis," 129

Baboons, 201–204
Behavioral and Brain Sciences, 164,
  165
Beldibi Cave, 187
Benyon, A. D., 14
Berenbaum, Sheri, 113
Bering land bridge, 173
Biological weapons, 195
Bipedalism, 13, 14, 80–100
  arboreal theory, 80–81, 230
  arboreal vestiges, 97–99
  brain evolution and, 4, 89, 159,
    162–163
  controversy over hominid, 3,
    80–100
  cranial blood flow and, 133–135,
    159–160, 163, 168
  female sexuality and theories of,
    92
  "flasher" theories, 92–94
  food acquisition theories, 89–91
  hunting and, 89
  knuckle-walking hypothesis, 82–84
  Laetoli footprints, 4, 27, 85–88
  man-the-gatherer hypothesis, 91
  radiator theory and, 4, 7, 94–97,
    160–165, 168
  sexual selection, 92–93
  sketch of earliest bipedal ancestors,
    97–99
  "2001" model, 88–89, 90
  woman-the-gatherer hypothesis, 90–
    91, 92
Birds, brain lateralization of, 121
Black Skull, 19–20, 137–139, 141,
  151, 166–167
Body fat, loss of, 162, 168
Body language, 71–74, 109, 202
Body parts, inability to identify as
  one's own, 67
Boesch, Christophe, 57
Boesch, Hedwige, 57

Bonobos (pygmy chimpanzees), 57, 244–245
  locomotion by, 82–83
  theory of common ancestor resembling, 82–84
Brace, C. Loring, 172, 241
Brain, Dr. C. K. (Bob), 30, 222
Braindance, 173–197
  defined, 173
Brain lateralization, 5, 75, 101–123
  in animals other than humans, 117–119
  evolution of, 5, 119–122, 176–177, 183
  lateralization research, 102–105, 107
  left hemisphere, *see* Left hemisphere of the brain
  mind-body problem, 107–109
  prenatal chemical environment and, 106–107, 114–115, 176–177
  research on commissurotomy patients, 102–104, 107–109
  right hemisphere, *see* Right hemisphere of the brain
  sexual differences, 5, 109–117
  sexual dimorphism in patterns of, 110–112
  timing of brain development and, 7, 107, 176
Brain shape, 112
Brain size:
  of australopithecines, 32, 76, 163
  of chimpanzees, 43, 76
  of *Homo*, 43, 81
  of *Homo habilis*, 144, 145
  of *Homo sapiens*, 171
  increase in, 30–32, 89
    bipedalism and, 4, 89, 159, 162–163
    of genus *Homo*, 4, 6, 50, 96–97, 144, 163, 169, 173, 175, 177–180, 184
    intelligence and, 178, 180, 188
    radiator network of veins and, 159, 163, 173
    suggested reasons for, 178–180

tool production and, 89
  sexual dimorphism in, 110
Brain temperature, regulation of, 27, 156–159
  increase in brain size and, 159, 163, 173
Brinnel, Heiner, 156–158
Broca, Paul, 68–69
Broca's aphasia, 69
Broca's area, 48–49, 68–71, 73–74, 176, 225
  in early *Homo*, 50, 169–170, 183
Brodman's areas, 225
Bromage, Tim, 14, 48
Broom, Mary, 20
Broom, Robert, 15–17, 20
Burial of the dead, 182
Bush, George, 216–217

Cabanac, Michel, 156–159
Calendars, 185
Calvin, William, 242
Cannibalism, 171, 172, 182–183, 201, 205, 242–243
Capuchin monkey, 57
Cave art, 173, 184, 188, 191–192
Cerebral cortex:
  of australopithecines, 4
  of chimpanzees, 5
  evolution of, in *Homo*, 50
  of *Homo*, 5, 50–51, 59–63, 175, 176, 177
Chagnon, Napoleon, 213
Cheverud, Jim, 41–42
Chimpanzees:
  aggression, 25, 200–201, 204–211
  cerebral cortex of, 5, 59–63
  common ancestor with humans, *see* Common ancestor (CA) of humans and chimpanzees
  comparison of brains of humans and of, 45, 58–76
    association cortices, 66–68
    cerebral cortex, 59–63
    frontal lobes, 63–66
    language abilities, 68–74
    with Taung endocast, 44–46

Chimpanzees *(cont'd)*
  diet of, 23
  inability to plan ahead, 57, 65
  intelligence of, 58
  knuckle-walking by, 23
  lack of awareness of death, 57, 65
  language abilities, 54–57
  life-style of, 23–25
  self-recognition of, 25, 53–54, 180
  sexual dimorphism of, 23–25
  sexuality of, 23
  simultaneous tasks, inability to per-
    form, 57, 65
  social interaction by, 25
  territoriality of, 25, 211
  tools and, 25
Circling behavior, 118–119, 120
Cladistic analysis, 3, 139–141, 151
Clarke, Ron, 167
Cohn, B. A., 161
Commissurotomy, 102–104, 107
Common ancestor (CA) of humans and
    chimpanzees, 211, 230
  as arboreal, 80–81
  as knuckle-walker, 82–84
  social behavior of, 97
Comprehension of language, 69,
  70
Congenital adrenal hyperphasia
  (CAH), 113–114
Conroy, Glenn, 14, 48, 133–135,
  136, 152
Consciousness, 108–109
Construct, ability to, 57–58
Contralateral rule, 61, 102–103
Coppens, Y., 131, 132, 136
Corpus callosum, 75, 235
  severing of, 102
Counting, 71, 185–186
Cranial blood flow, 132–137,
  152–165
  brain temperature and, 156–159,
    163, 173
  evolution of, 153–155, 168, 177,
    240
  posture and, 133–135, 159–160,
    163, 168

  see also Occipital/marginal (O/M)
    sinus
Creationists, 78
Cro-Magnon, 173, 188–192
Curiosity, 81, 178

Daly, Martin, 214–216
Dart, Raymond, 2, 9–13, 35
  Taung fossil, 2, 9–13, 20
    humanlike features stressed by, 2,
      4, 10, 12–13, 21, 32–34
Darwin, Charles, 1, 78, 79
Darwinian theory, 78, 79
Dean, Christopher, 14
Death, awareness of, 57, 65, 179,
  181–183
Defense Mobilization Planning Sys-
    tems Agency, 216–217
Dentition:
  of australopithecines, 13, 14, 26
    gracile, 18, 167–168
    robust, 18
  of gorillas, 22–23
  of *Homo habilis*, 144, 145, 148
  of Lucy's child, 148
De Waal, Frans, 208–209, 244–245
Dexterity skills, 117
Diet:
  of chimpanzees, 23
  of gorillas, 22–23
  of gracile australopithecines, 18–
    19, 26, 28
  of robust australopithecines, 18–19,
    26, 160, 166
Dominance hierarchies and aggres-
    sion, 201–204, 208
Dopamine, 107, 113, 118, 176
Doppler probe, 157
Dyslexia, 115

Eastern highland gorilla, 22
Eberhard, William C., 232
Emissary veins, 153, 156–158, 240
Emotions, 7, 66
  control of, 195–197
  left hemisphere of the brain and,
    105

Emotions *(cont'd)*
  right hemisphere of the brain and, 104, 105–106
Endocasts (fossil skulls), 4
ER 405, 129, 167
ER 1470, 169, 183, 184
ER 1805, 168
ER 3733, 129
Eskimos, 212, 213
Essay on the Principle of Population, An (Malthus), 78–79
Estrogen, 112–113, 114
Estrus, 23, 202
Eve hypothesis, 241
Extraterrestrial intelligence, 247

Faces, recognition of, 106
Family trees:
  based on molecules, 78
  cladistic analysis, 139–141, 151
  fossil-based, 77
  hominid, 165–173
  mix-up in hominid, 125–150
    cranial blood flow evidence, 132–137
    discovery of the Black Skull and, 137–139, 151
    naming of *Australopithecus afarensis*, 129, 131
    OH 62 and, 147–150
Female-male differences, *see* Sexual dimorphism
Females in dominance hierarchy, 202–4
Finding the Missing Link (Broom), 15
Fire, 170–171, 222
FitzGerald, Randall, 120–121
Foramina in the skull, 153–154, 240
Fossils:
  family trees based on, 77
  hominid fossil record, 2, 81, 84–85, 99–100, 145–150, 153, 166, 167, 169, 171, 173, 224, 233
  Hadar, *see* Hadar, Ethiopia, fossils from
  Laetoli, 4, 27, 85–88, 128, 129, 167, 168, 231

Frontal lobes, 61, 63–66, 145
  Broca's area, *see* Broca's area convolution of, 47
  human vs. chimpanzee, 65
Functional morphology, 3
Fusion-fission society, 23

Galaburda, Albert, 114–115
Gallup, Gordon, 25, 53–54, 180, 181
Gardner, Allen, 54
Gardner, Beatrice, 54, 178
Gaulin, Steven, 120–121
Gebusi of New Guinea, 212–214
Gender, *see* Sexual dimorphism
Gene frequencies, 229
Genome Project, 194–195
Geschwind, Norman, 114–115
Gesticulation, *see* Body language
Gibson, Kathleen, 57–58, 178
Glick, Stanley, 117–120, 176
Goldin-Meadow, Susan, 73
Goldman-Rakie, Patricia, 64, 65
Gombe National Park, 25, 204
Goodall, Jane, 25, 93, 204–205, 210, 211, 220
Gorillas:
  diet of, 22–23
  harem social life of, 22–23
  knuckle-walking by, 23
  life-style of, 21–23
  sexual dimorphism, 23
Gracile australopithecines, 169
  characteristics of, 17
  cranial blood flow in, 154, 155, 160
  diet of, 18–19, 26, 28
  discovery of, 15
  from East Africa, 50
  on family tree, 166
  habitat of, 27
  life-style of, 26, 27–28
  naming of, 15
  O/M sinus in, 154, 155, 168
  sexual dimorphism of, 28
  social life of, 28
  tool use by, 19
Grooming, 22, 197
Grün, Ranier, 172

Hadar, Ethiopia, fossils from, 36, 126, 128, 129, 160, 167
  as ancestral to robust australopithecines, 135, 137, 143
  differences in, attributed to sex, 129, 131, 142
  on family tree, 167–168
  O/M sinus in, 133, 135, 136–137, 142–143, 152
Hair loss, 161, 162, 168
Hampson, Elizabeth, 112
Handedness, 105, 118, 121–122
  brain shape and, 112
  see also Left-handers; Right-handers
Harems, 22–23, 27
Hearing, 61, 62, 67, 68
Height of *Homo erectus*, 145–146, 170
Hildebolt, Charles (Scooter), 40, 41–46
Hines, Melissa, 113, 114, 118
Hippocampus, 196
Holloway, Ralph, 13, 34–37, 43, 152, 165, 222, 238
Hominidae:
  bipedalism, *see* Bipedalism
  family tree, *see* Family trees
  fossil record, *see* Fossils
  sexuality of, 92
  see also specific genuses and species
Hominid paleontologists:
  bipedalism controversy, *see* Bipedalism
  disagreement among, 2–3
  limited access to fossils, 3, 4, 28–29, 222
Homo, 4, 50, 142
  beliefs about ancestors of, 19
  brain lateralization, *see* Brain lateralization
  brain size increase in, 4, 6, 50, 96–97, 144, 169, 175, 177–180, 184
  cranial radiator system and, 163, 173
  intelligence and, 178, 180, 188

cerebral cortex of, 5, 50–51, 59–63, 175, 176
chimpanzee brain and brain of, *see* Chimpanzees, comparison of brains of humans and of
common ancestor, *see* Common ancestor (CA) of humans and chimpanzees
cranial blood flow's evolution, 154–155, 168, 177
distinguishing characteristics, 145, 169–170
family tree, 77–78, 166, 169–173
O/M sinus of, 135, 153
sexual dimorphism in brain of, 102
shifts in timing of development of parts of the brain and, 6–7
see also Homo erectus; Homo habilis; Homo sapiens
Homicide, 212–216
Homicide (Daly and Wilson), 215
Homo erectus, 50, 143, 170–171, 183
  brain size, 170
  family tree, 169
  fossil record, 145–146, 149, 169, 171, 224
  life-style of, 170–171
Homo habilis, 50, 143–145, 148, 183
  brain size of, 144, 145
  dentition of, 144
  family tree, 169
  fossil record of, 143–144, 168, 169, 224
  naming of, 144
Homo sapiens, 50, 150, 171–173, 241
  brain size of, 171
  cranial blood flow in, 153, 155
  distinguishing characteristics, 171
  family tree, 169
  Laetoli hominid footprints and, 85–88
  migration of, 193
Homunculus, 59–61, 224–25
Hormones, sex, 112–119
Howell, Clark, 142
Hrdy, Sarah Blaffer, 244

Humor, 106
Hunting, 90, 170, 173, 193
  group, 204–205
Hydrostatic pressure, 134

Idiopathic hypogonadotrophic hypo-
    gonadism, 114
Imagination, 66
Intelligence:
  brain size and, 178, 180, 188
  of chimpanzees versus humans, 58
*International Code of Zoological No-
    menclature,* 129–130, 131

Jerison, Harry, 46, 48, 61, 178, 184
Johanson, Donald, 143
  discovery of Lucy, 92, 126
  Lucy's Child, 135–136, 137
  Lucy's child and, 147–148
  naming of *Australopithecus afar-
    ensis,* 128, 129, 132, 142
Journal of Human Evolution, 131
Jungers, Bill, 14, 48

Kalahari San, *see* !Kung
Kanzi (chimpanzee), 55–57
Kasinga, Simon, 50
Kendon, Adam, 71–72, 73
Kerr, Richard, 247
Killing, 200, 201, 204
  homicide, 212–216
Kimbel, William, 136, 142, 165
Kimura, Doreen, 111, 112, 178
Kirtlandia, 131
Kluver-Bucy syndrome, 68
Knapp, Bob, 40
Knauft, Bruce, 212–214
KNM-ER 406, 129, 167
KNM-ER 1470, 50, 51, 144–145
KNM-ER 3733, 129
KNM-WT 15000, *see* Turkana Boy
KNM-WT 17000, *see* WT 17000
Knuckle-walking, 23, 82–84, 230
Kohler, Wolfgang, 180
Kromdraai, South Africa, 15–17
!Kung, 200, 212, 213

Laetoli, Tanzania, fossils from, 128,
    129, 142
  differences in attributed to sex, 129
  Laetoli footprints, 4, 27, 85–88,
    142, 167, 168, 231
  O/M sinus in, 142
Lake Turkana, Kenya, fossils from,
    144, 145, 146, 149, 169
Lamboid suture of the skull, 33
  confused with lunate sulcus of the
    brain, 33
  Falk-Holloway dispute, 34–37
Language, 6, 50, 105, 183–188, 220
  age and ability to learn foreign, 56,
    74, 194
  art and, 189–190
  beginnings of, 184–185
  body language, 71–74, 109, 202
  chimpanzees ability to learn non-
    verbal, 54–57
  comprehension of, 69, 70
  development of distinct languages,
    193
  sensory and motor components of,
    69
  sexual dimorphism in language
    skills, 109, 117
  speech, *see* Speech
  writing, 6, 185–188, 193
Language Research Center, 57
Lascaux cave art, 191–192
Lateralization, *see* Brain lateraliza-
    tion
Leakey, Louis, 49, 144, 169
Leakey, Mary, 4, 95, 178
  fossilized footprints discovered by,
    4, 27, 85
Leakey, Richard, 49, 129, 132, 143,
    145, 222
Left-handers, 105, 112, 115, 190
Left hemisphere of the brain, 61, 69–
    70, 71
  contralateral rule, 61, 102–103
  development of, 71, 107, 114–115,
    176
  functions of, 105, 108, 234
  see also Brain lateralization

LeMay, Marjorie, 112, 178
Lewin, Roger, 191–192
L.H.-21, 168
Limbic system, 7, 66, 196–197, 219, 220
Lobotomies, prefrontal, 63
Lorenz, Konrad, 199–200
Lovejoy, Owen, 13, 91, 92
Lucy (fossil), 3, 92, 125–128, 142, 143
   "child" of, 147–150
   described, 126–128
   discovery of, 126
Lucy's Child (Johanson), 135–136
Lucy's child (OH 62), 147–150
Lunate sulcus of the brain, 223
   computer measurement of, 40, 42
   confused with lamboid suture of the skull, 33–34
      Falk-Holloway dispute, 34–37
   in humans, 33–34, 61–62
   in Taung fossil, 34, 48

Macaques, 121
   prefrontal cortex of, 64
McDonnell Douglas 3Space Digitizer (3Space), 40, 46
MacNeilage, Peter, 121–122
Makapansgat, South Africa, fossils from, 131
Male-female differences, *see* Sexual dimorphism
Mallinckrodt Institute of Radiology, Washington University Medical Center, 39
Malthus, Thomas Robert, 78–79, 229–230
Man-the-gatherer hypothesis, 91
Maser, Jack, 180, 181
Mastoid emissary veins, 153, 156–158
Mastoid foramina, 154
Matata (chimpanzee), 55, 56
Mathematics skills, sexual dimorphism in, 109
Mead, Margaret, 200

Memories, 196
   accessing and keeping, on-line, 64, 65
Mendel, Gregor, 79
Metaphor, ability to understand, 106
Missing links, 1, 12
Molecular anthropologists, 78, 79–80, 241
Monogamy, 92, 197
Mosaic evolution, 231
Mothering, 81
Motor area of the brain, *see* Primary motor area of the brain
Multiple tasks, performing, 57, 65
Musical abilities, 105, 108, 109–110, 234
Mutations, 78

Naming of new zoological species, 129–132, 144
   splitters, 15, 19–20
   see also specific species
National Museum of Kenya, 49–50
Natural selection, 78, 79, 176, 177, 178–179
Nature, 12, 129, 131, 135
Neandertals, 171–172, 181–182
Nervous system, 5
Norepinephrine, 107
Nuclear weapons, 195, 216–219, 246–247
Nunn, Sam, 218–219

Occipital association cortex, 66–67
Occipital/marginal (O/M) sinus, 132–137, 152–155, 238
   function of, 132–133
   in gracile australopithecines, 154, 155, 168
   in humans, 135, 153
   in robust australopithecines, 133, 135, 137, 154, 155, 163, 166, 238
Offutt, Carolyn, 40
OH 62 (Lucy's child), 147–150
Olduvai Gorge, 19, 143, 144, 147

Olduwan pebble tools, 19
Olfactory associations, *see* Smell, sense of
Olson, Todd, 137
Omo region, Ethiopia, fossils from, 144
O/M sinus, *see* Occipital/marginal (O/M) sinus
On Aggression (Lorenz), 199
On the Origin of Species by Means of Natural Selection. . . (Darwin), 1, 79
Orangutans, 57, 230
"Out of Africa" theory, 241

Paleoanthropologists, 77–78, 241
    bipedalism dispute, *see* Bipedalism
    resistance to new hypotheses, 82, 164
    selective interpretation of evidence by, 13, 21
Paleontologists, hominid, *see* Hominid paleontologists *Paranthropus robustus*, 17
    see also Robust australopithecines
Parietal association cortex, 66–67
Parietal emissary veins, 153, 156–158
Parietal foramina, 154
Parietal lobe, 61
Patas monkeys, 162
Patrolling behavior, 210–211, 216–219
Peacemaking Among Primates (De Waal), 208–209
Peacemaking behavior, 209
Pebble tools, 19
Peer review, 130–131, 164–165
Peking Man, 171
Penfield, Wilder, 59
Penises, 93, 232
Personality, prefrontal association cortex and, 63
Petalias, 112, 235
Pfeiffer, John, 173
Phoenicians, 187
Pictographs, 186, 187
Planning ability, 57, 64, 65, 179, 180

Play, 81
Population management, 195, 243
Prefrontal association cortex, 63–66, 176, 177, 180
Premotor cortex, 62, 65
Primary auditory cortex, 61, 62
Primary motor area of the brain, 59, 73–74
    body parts represented on, 59–61
    linkage with premotor cortex, 62
Primary somatosensory area of the brain, 59–62
    body parts represented on, 59–61
    linkage with association cortex, 62
Primary visual cortex, 62
Primate evolution, 77
Progesterone, 112–113
Proper mass, principle of, 61
Pygmy chimpanzees, *see* Bonobos

Radiator theory, 4, 7, 94–97, 152–165, 168, 173, 177
Radinsky, Leonard, 33, 34
rain lateralization:
    evolution of, 5, 119–122, 176–177, 183
Rats, 117–118
Reagan, Ronald, 218
Red Cave, 28–33, 222
Reed, Charles, 30
Religion, 181–183
Rhesus monkeys, 40–43, 115–116
Richards, Graham, 97–99
Riffle, Cynthia, 74–75, 226–229
Right-handers, 112, 170, 183
Right hemisphere of the brain, 75
    contralateral rule, 61, 102–103
    development of, 107, 114–115, 176
    functions of, 104, 105–106, 121
    see also Brain lateralization
Robinson, John, 17–19, 20, 60
Robust australopithecines:
    Australopithecus afarensis as ancestors of, 135, 137, 143
    Black Skull, *see* Black Skull
    characteristics of, 17

Robust australopithecines *(cont'd)*
  diet of, 18–19, 26, 160, 166
  discovery of, 15–17
  from East Africa, 49–50, 160, 166–167
  on family tree, 166
  habitat of, 26
  life-style of, 26–27
  naming of, 17
  O/M sinus in, 133, 135, 137, 154, 155, 163, 166, 238
  sexual dimorphism of, 26
  tool use by, 27, 222
Rod-and-frame test, 113
Rumbaugh, Dennis, 55

Salmons, Josephine, 9
Savage-Rumbaugh, Sue, 55, 57, 58, 65, 178
Schmandt-Besserat, Denise, 178, 185–187, 193
Science, 118, 131, 132
Scopes, John, 2, 12
Self, sense of, 104, 180
Self-recognition by chimpanzees, 25, 53–54
Semai of Malaya, 212, 213
Senses:
  primary somatosensory area of the brain, 59–61
  see also specific senses
Senut, Brigitte, 13–14, 137, 142, 178
Seville Statement on Violence, 245–246
Sex hormones, 112–119
Sexism, 3, 201–204
Sexual competition, 200, 208, 210, 213
Sexual dimorphism:
  in brain size, 110
  of chimpanzees, 23–25
  of gorillas, 23
  of gracile australopithecines, 28
  of human brain, 5, 102, 109–117, 122, 234
  in language skills, 109

  of robust australopithecines, 26
  in visuospatial skills, 67–68, 109, 110, 112
Sexuality:
  of chimpanzees, 23
  of early hominids, 92, 93, 97
  of gorillas, 22
  sexual selection of males, 92–93, 232
Shadow (chimpanzee), 93
Shanidar Cave, 182
Shipman, Pat, 65, 178
Single-species hypothesis, 129
Skelton, Randall, 141
Skilled movement, left hemisphere of brain and, 105
Smell, sense of, 196
  hallucinations, 68
Smith, Holly, 14, 48, 178
Social behavior, 178–179
  of apes, 22–23, 25
  of common ancestor, 97
  frontal lobe and human, 66
  of gracile australopithecines, 28
  limbic system and, 197
  of robust australopithecines, 27
Social intelligence, 178–179, 180–181
Spatial skills, *see* Visuospatial skills
Speech, 177, 179, 184–185, 187–188
  body language and, 71–74
  Broca's area, 48–49, 68–71, 73–74
Sperry, Roger, 102–104, 108–109
Splitters, 15, 19–20, 142, 165
State University of New York at Albany, 53
Strapping Youth, *see* Turkana Boy
Strategic Integrated Operations Plan (SIOP-7), 218
Stringer, Christopher, 172, 241
Stuttering, 115
Sumerians, 186–187
Summers, Harry G., Jr., 246–247
Sweat glands, 161, 162, 168
Swift, Jonathan, 230
Swiss Center for Scientific Research, 57

Sylvian fissure, 61

Taieb, Maurice, 128
Tanner, Nancy, 92–93
Tap dancing, 65, 74–76, 226–229
Tardieu, Christine, 137, 142
Taung fossil, 2, 9–13, 20–21, 44–48,
    133, 160
  comparison with brain of a human
    child and a chimpanzee, 44–46
  digitalized measurement of, 43–44,
    46
  discovery of, 2
  humanlife features stressed, 2, 4,
    10, 12–13, 21, 32–34
  lamboid suture of skull confused
    with lunate sulcus of the brain,
    33–34
    Falk-Holloway dispute, 34–37
  location of, 32
  proven through measurement to be
    apelike, 44–47
Teeth, *see* Dentition
Temperature:
  brain, *see* Brain temperature
  radiator theory, 4, 7, 94–97, 160–
    165, 168
Temporal association cortex, 66–67,
    68
Temporal lobe of the brain, 61
Terblanche, Gert, 15
Territorial Imperative, The (Ardrey),
    199
Territoriality, 200, 219, 220
  of chimpanzees, 25, 211
  patrolling, 210–211, 216–219
Testosterone, 114, 115
3Space, *see* McDonnell Douglas
    3Space Digitizer
Time:
  binding of, 66, 179
  counting, 71, 185–186
  left hemisphere of the brain and,
    105, 179
Tobias, Phillip, 20, 32, 45, 50, 132,
    145, 170, 222, 238
Tools, 170

brain size and production of, 89
chimpanzees and, 25
gracile australopithecine's use of,
    19
human's unique use of, 57
of late Stone Age, 173
of Neandertals, 172
robust australopithecine's use of,
    27, 221–222
Toth, Nick, 170
Touch, 67
Transvaal Museum, 19
  Red Cave, 28–33, 222
"Treetop," 216, 217, 218
Turkana Boy (WT 15000), 143, 145–
    146, 149, 169
Turner syndrome, 114
Tuttle, Russell, 85, 137, 142, 165,
    168, 231
"2001" model, 88–89, 90

University of Witwatersrand, 32
Upper-Paleolithic art, 188–192

Vannier, Michael, 14, 37, 39–41, 43,
    48
Vegetarianism:
  of gorillas, 22–23
  of robust australopithecines, 18, 26,
    160, 166
Vertebral plexis, 135
  see also Cranial blood flow
Violence, *see* Aggression
Vision, 61–62, 68
  hallucinations, 68
  inability to interpret visual output,
    67
Visuospatial skills, 67, 120–121
  right hemisphere of the brain and,
    105
  sex hormones and, 113, 114
  sexual dimorphism in, 67–68, 109,
    110, 112
Voles, 120–121
Vrba, Elizabeth, 30, 160, 178

Walker, Alan, 129, 132, 145

Wallace, Alfred Russell, 78, 79
Ward, Jeannette, 101
Washburn, Sherwood, 231
Washoe (chimpanzee), 54
Wernicke's aphasia, 69
Wernicke's area, 69, 70, 225
Wheeler, Pete, 94–97, 99, 161–162, 163
White, Tim, 128, 131, 132, 136, 137, 142, 167
Wilberforce, Mrs., 1–2
Wilson, Margo, 214–216
Woman-the-gatherer hypothesis, 90–91
Women, *see* Sexual dimorphism

Wrangham, Richard, 97
Writing, 6, 185–188, 193
WT 15000, *see* Turkana Boy
WT 17000 (Black Skull), 19–20, 137–139, 141, 151, 166–167
Wynn, Thomas, 122

Yanomamo, 213–14
Yerkese (language), 55
Yerkes Regional Primate Center, 55

Zansky, Michael, 192
Zihlman, Adrienne, 81–82, 91, 92, 137, 142, 161, 178
Zimmerberg, Betty, 118, 178